Chromosomal Abnormalities

Edited by Tülay Aşkın Çelik and Subrata Dey

Published in London, United Kingdom

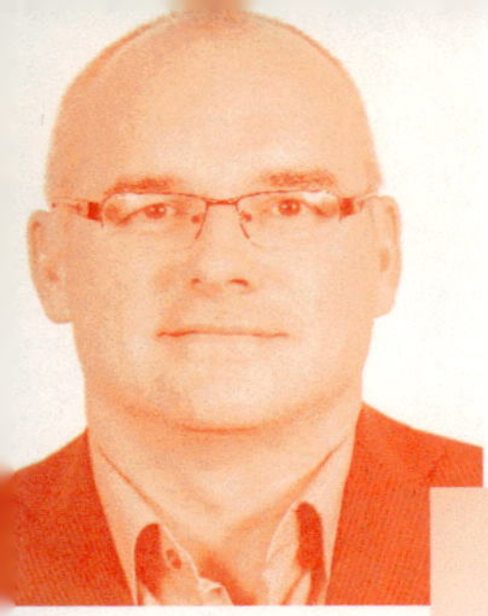
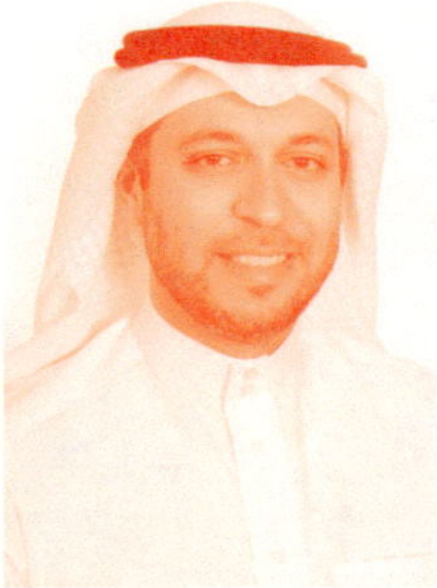
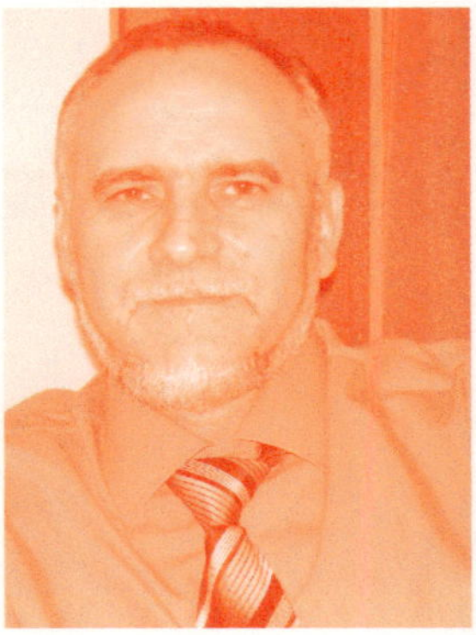
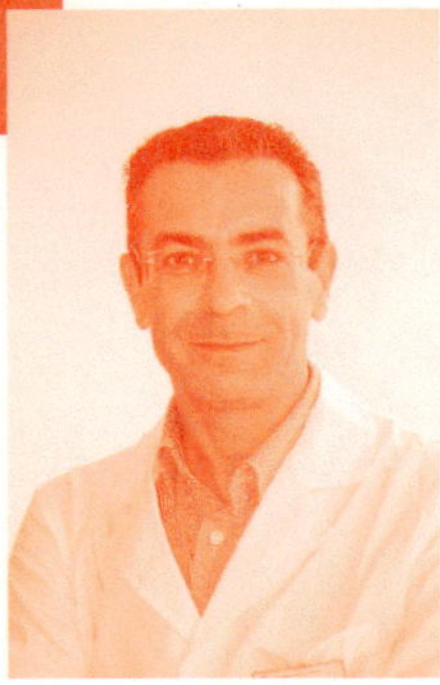
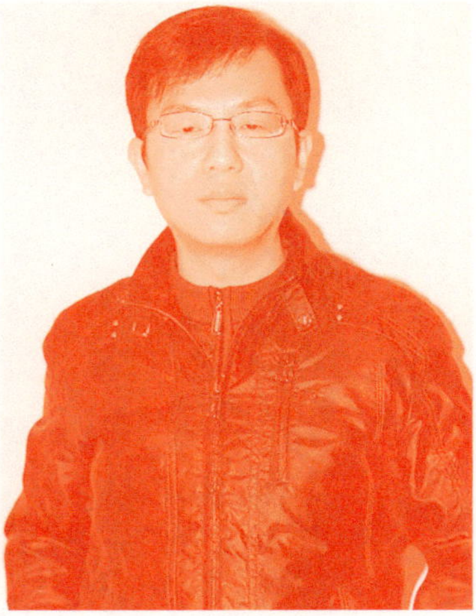
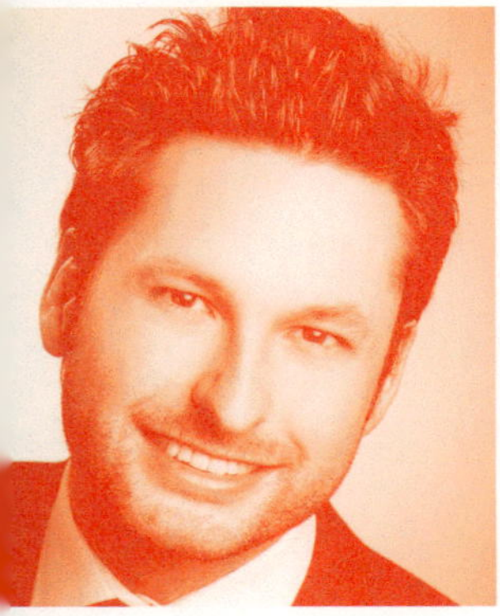
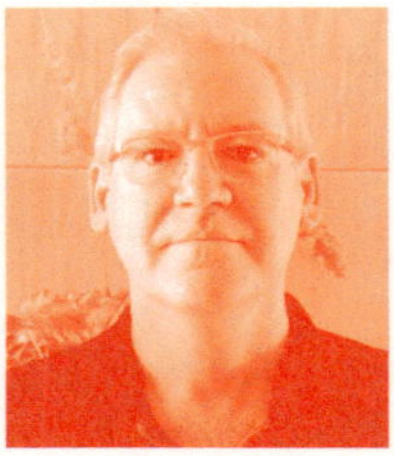

IntechOpen

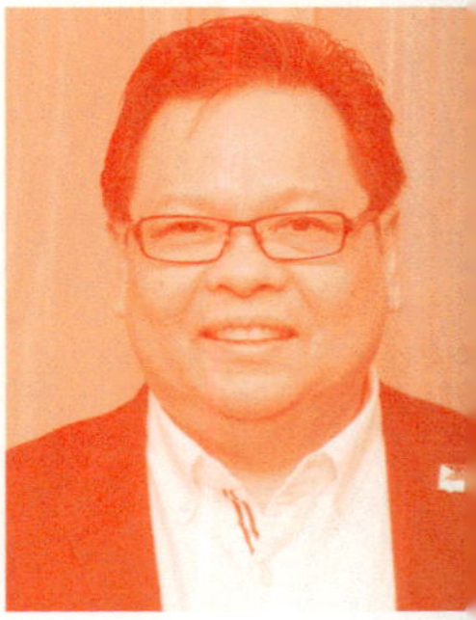
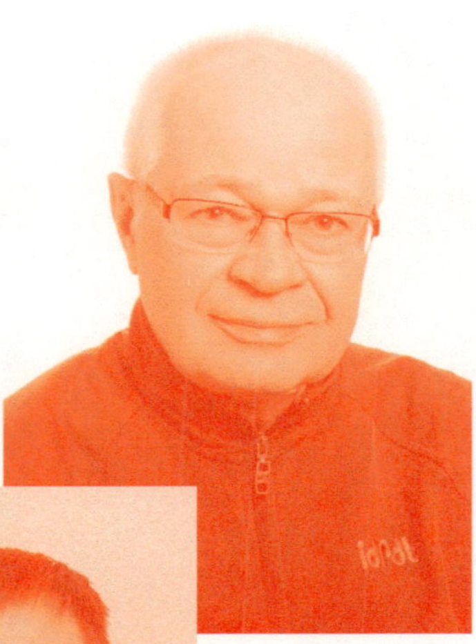
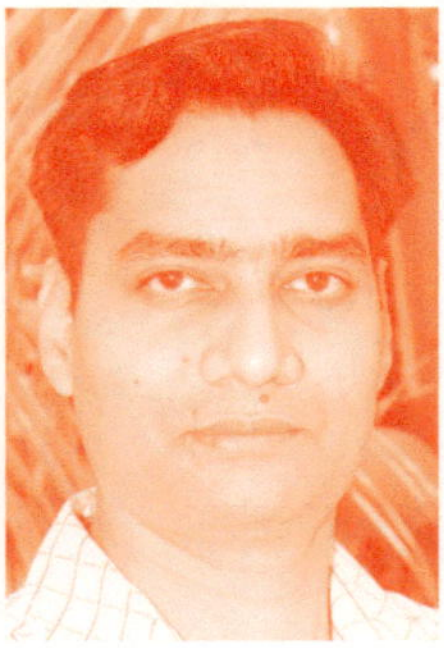
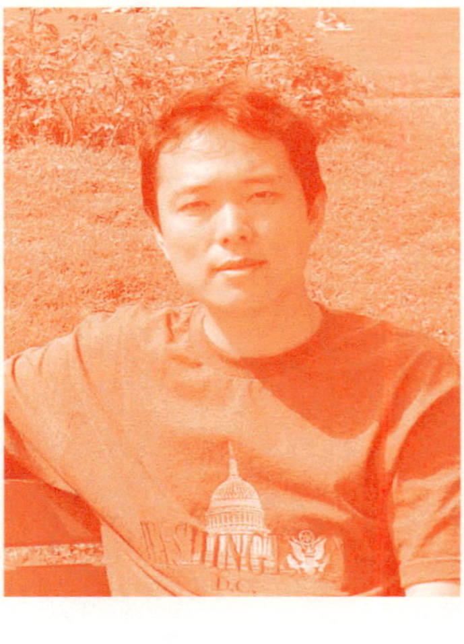
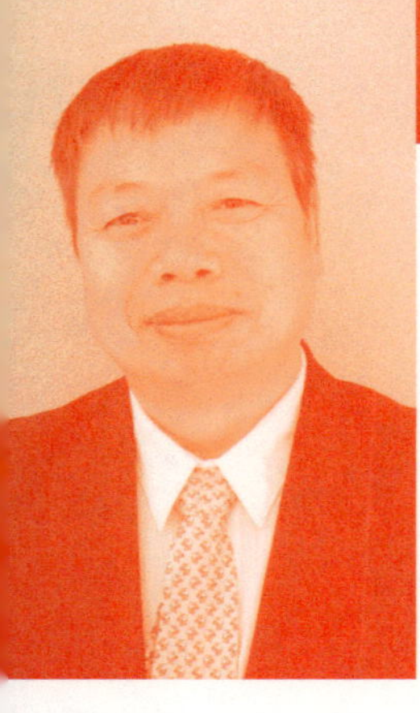
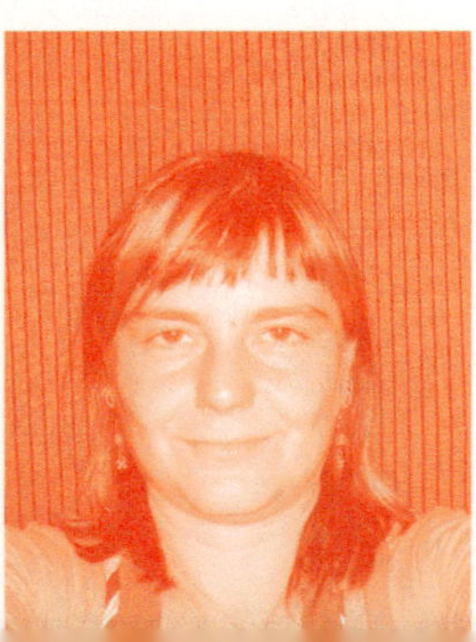

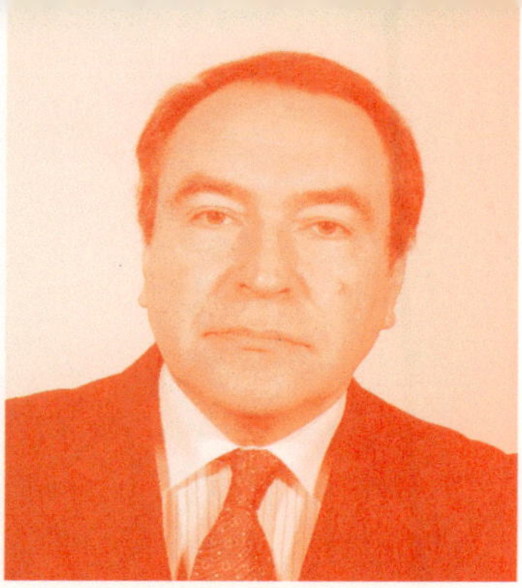
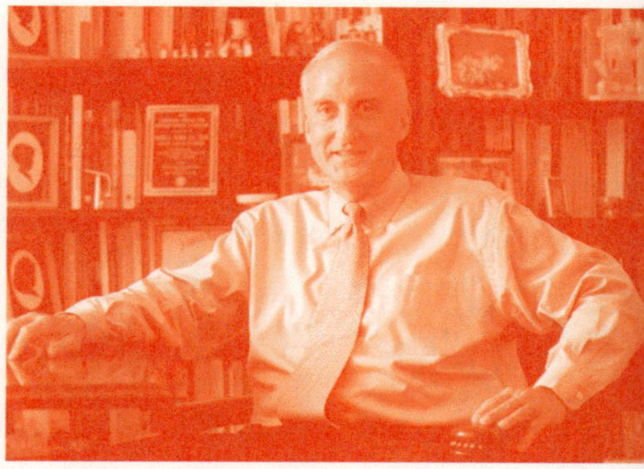
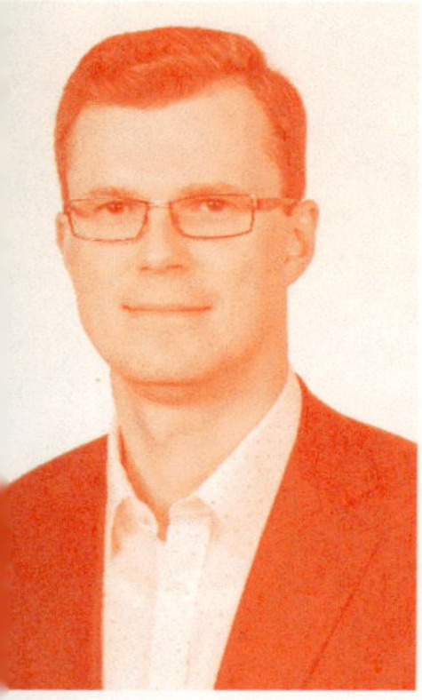
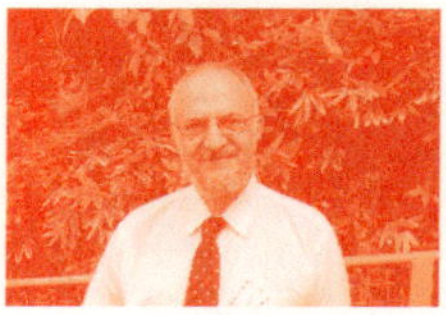
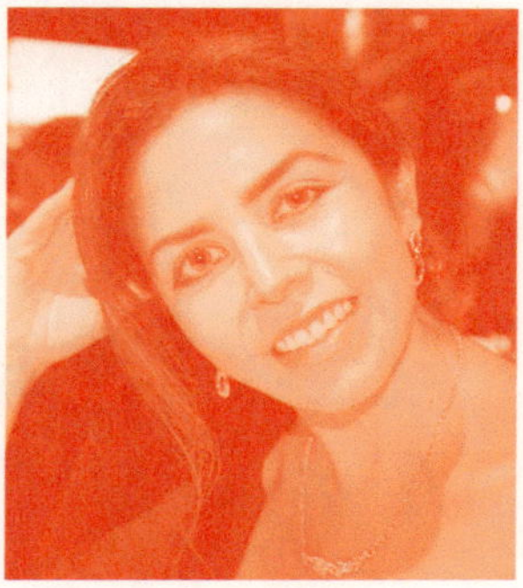

Supporting open minds since 2005

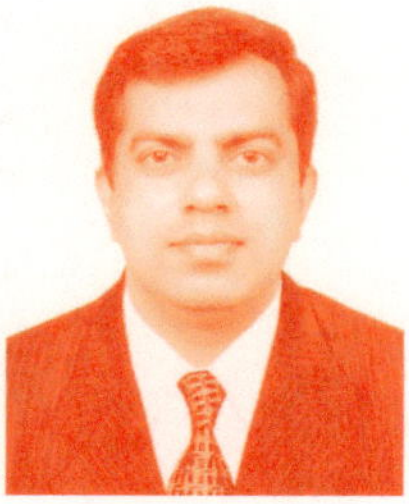
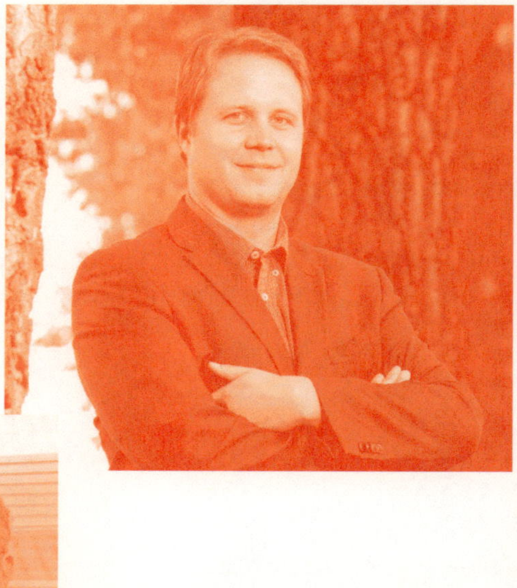
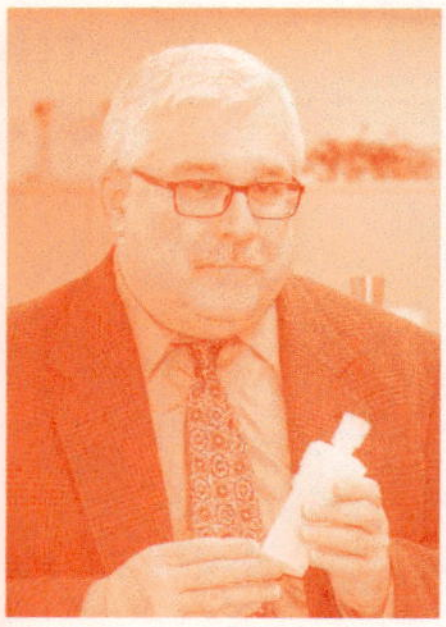
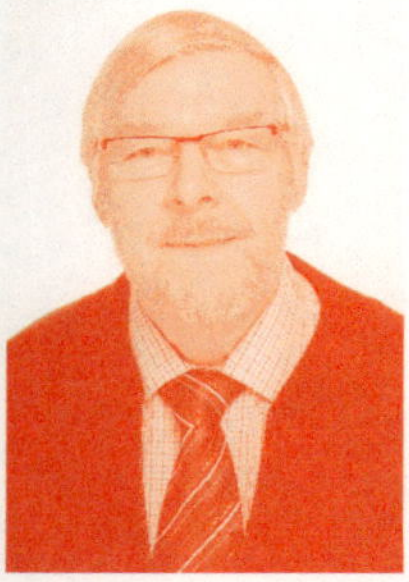
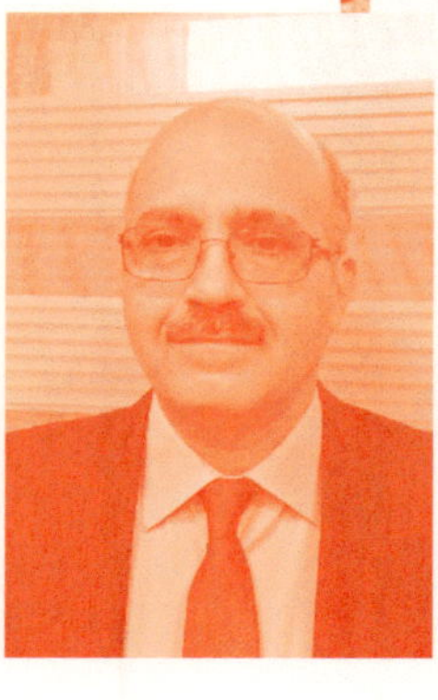
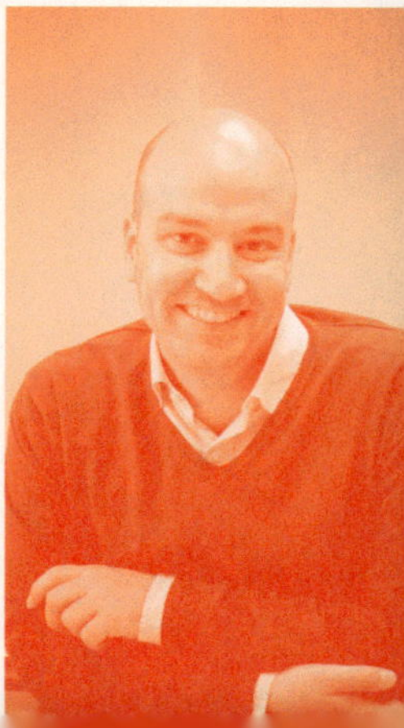
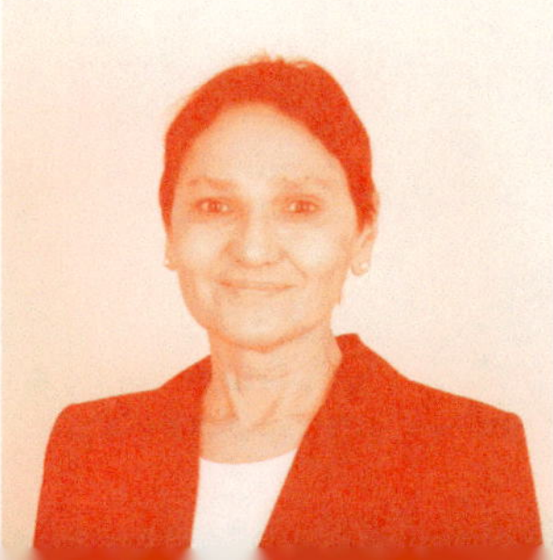

Chromosomal Abnormalities
http://dx.doi.org/10.5772/intechopen.77904
Edited by Tülay Aşkın Çelik and Subrata Dey

Contributors
Artúr Beke, Aténé Simonyi, Sujay Ghosh, Papiya Ghosh, Kesara Anamthawat-Jónsson, Puangpaka Umpunjun, Aurora Arghir, Magdalena Budisteanu, Andreea Tutulan-Cunita, Ina Focsa, Sorina Mihaela Papuc, Mounia Bendari, Nisrine Khoubila, Siham Cherkaoui, Mouna Lamhahab, Meryem Qachouh, Nezha Hda, Asmaa Quessar, Margarida L. R. Aguiar-Perecin, Mateus Mondin, José Raulindo Gardingo, Janay A. Santos-Serejo, Subrata Kumar Dey, Arturo Solis Herrera, Tülay Aşkın Çelik, Pranami Bhaumik, Mandar Bhattacharya

First published in London, United Kingdom, 2020 by IntechOpen
IntechOpen is the global imprint of INTECHOPEN LIMITED, registered in England and Wales, registration number: 11086078, 5 Princes Gate Court, London, SW7 2QJ, United Kingdom
Printed in Croatia

British Library Cataloguing-in-Publication Data
A catalogue record for this book is available from the British Library

Additional hard and PDF copies can be obtained from orders@intechopen.com

Chromosomal Abnormalities
Edited by Tülay Aşkın Çelik and Subrata Dey
p. cm.
Print ISBN 978-1-78985-979-9
Online ISBN 978-1-78985-980-5
eBook (PDF) ISBN 978-1-83968-978-9

For EU product safety concerns:
IN TECH d. o. o., Prolaz Marije Krucifikse Kozulić 3, 51000 Rijeka, Croatia, info@intechopen.com or visit our website at intechopen.com.

Meet the editors

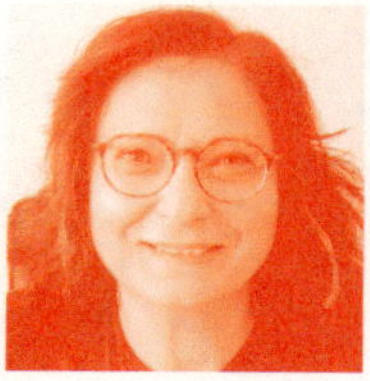

Dr. Tülay Aşkın Çelik gained her PhD from Fırat University, Art and Science Faculty, Department of Biology, Elazığ/TURKEY. Presently she is an Associate Professor at Aydın Adnan Menderes University, Art and Science Faculty, Department of Biology, Aydın/TURKEY in the field of genetics. She has been a referee for more than 25 international scientific journals and she worked as a researcher and project manager in 13 projects. She is a referent for issues related to the fields of genetic toxicology and anticancer and antioxidant plants. In 2008, she became a member of the European Association for Cancer Research (EACR) and Molecular Cancer Research Association (MOKAD) and in 2018, she became a member of the Medical Biology and Genetics Association (TBGDER). Currently, her scientific interests include bioactive phytochemicals and plant extracts on their cytogenetic and gentotoxic effects on chromosomes and cancer cells and in vivo /in vitro biological activities. Furthermore, she is also investigating the genotoxic and cytotoxic effects of environmental pollutants such as pesticides. She has authored one book and two book chapters in reputed books published by IntechOpen Access Publisher.

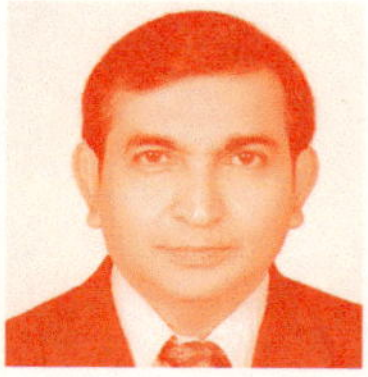

Prof. Subrata Dey received his Ph.D. degree from the University of Kalyani, India. He joined the faculty of Maulana Abul Kalam Azad University of Technology (formerly known as West Bengal University of Technology) as Professor of Biotechnology in 2005. His laboratory has long been involved in research on the molecular genetics of Down syndrome and other congenital disorders, the genetics of Alzheimer's disease, the genetics of congenital heart disease, radiation-induced genomic instability, radioprotection and stem cell biology. Prof. Dey received a Golden Jubilee Award for excellence in teaching and research. He has published more than 80 research papers in referred journals, edited five books on Down syndrome and has completed eleven research projects funded by the Government Of India. Several students also received their Ph.D. under his supervision. Along with teaching and research, Prof. Dey has handled a number of administrative assignments successfully and made dedicated and innovative approaches with great integrity. Major administrative roles were Director of School of Biotechnology and Biological Sciences, Founder Co-ordinator of Centre for Genetic Studies, Member-Coordinator of Ekta Incubation Centre, Pro-Vice Chancellor and Vice-Chancellor of Maulana Abul Kalam Azad University of Technology, Vice Chancellor of Brainware University. Recently he joined as Vice Chancellor of Swami Vivekananda University, West Bengal, India.

Contents

Preface

Cytogenetics is the study of chromosome structure and function in relation to phenotypic expression. Chromosomal defects underlie the development of a broad assortment of diseases and conditions ranging from Down syndrome to cancer and are of common concern in both fundamental and clinic research. Chromosomal defects are one of the most common causes of genetic disorders and are responsible for a large proportion of miscarriages. As a result, increasing numbers of parents are becoming interested in genetic counseling in order to learn about the risks of reproductive failure or to understand why they had a child with a particular defect, whether it will happen again, and what might have been done to prevent it. This book discusses the basic biological theory underlying chromosomal abnormalites and provides detalied information on the reproductive risks of chromosomally abnormal individuals and of normal parents.

Chromosome Abnormalities is a web-based resource that contains a series of chapters highlighting several aspects related to the generation of chromosomal abnormalities in genetic material. It is an essential resource for cytogeneticists, laboratory personnel, clinicians, research scientists, and students in the field. The book focuses on known or theorized issues directly related to chromosomal abnormalities observed in humans and plants in light of current scientific information in three separate parts: "Introduction", "Chromosomal Abnomalities Observed in Humans" and "Chromosomal Abnomalities Observed in Plants."

In the introductory chapter, Dr. Tülay Aşkın Çelik from Aydın, Turkey, defines, classifies, and provides general information about chromosomal anomalies and how they occur. In addition, the chapter examines the effects of structural and numerical changes in chromosomes, especially on human health. Finally, it emphasizes the importance of classical and molecular cytogenetic techniques in important potential applications, especially in clinical trials and biomedical diagnosis, comparing them against other molecular and genomic methods.

Chapter 2, "The risk a chromosomal abnormalities in cases of minor and major fetal anomalies in the second trimester," by Drs. Beke and Simonyi from Budapest, Hungary, describes the major and minor abnormalities that may occur in normal pregnancy, but that also increase the risk of certain chromosome aberrations. One of the most important techniques for diagnosing chromosomal abnormalities is the fetal ultrasound. In this chapter, researchers emphasize the importance of screening minor and major ultrasound abnormalities in detecting chromosomal abnormalities in the second trimester of pregnancy.

Chapter 3, "Impact of biological factors related to maternal aging: risk of childbirth with Down Syndrome," by Dr. Kumar Dey et al., from West Bengal, India, discusses how maternal aging and multiple biological factors, such as hormones, play a key role in Down syndrome. Hormonal dysfunction also affects the meiotic process and spindle structure integrity and contributes to chromosome nondisjunction. This chapter also discusses the association between maternal age, ovarian aging, environmental factors, and telomere shortening at older reproductive age and the birth of infants with trisomy 21 Down syndrome.

Chapter 4, Dr. Ghosh and Dr. Ghosh summarizes "Gene polymorphisms that predispose a women for Down syndrome childbirth," by Dr. Ghosh and Dr. Ghosh from West Bengal, India, summarizes the connection between Down syndrome childbirth and polymorphisms of the genes involved in chromosome division as well as recombination and folic acid metabolisms. They discuss and summarize studies conducted on different population samples from different parts of world to determine the common polymorphisms that can server as markers for preconceptional screening of Down syndrome risk among the women.

Chapter 5, "Current cytogenetic abnormalities in Acute Myeloid Leukemia (AML)," by Dr. Bendari et al. from Casablanca, Morocco, describes typical chromosomal abnormalities in AML. The authors use World Health Organization classifications of AML to adress gene mutations found in normal karyotype AML via cutting-edge, next-generation sequencing technologies such as FLT3-IT, NPM1, CEBPA, and other additional mutations.

Chapter 6, "First-tier array CGH in clinically variable entities diagnosis: 22q13.3 deletion syndrome," by Dr. Budisteanu et al. from Romania, summarizes Phelan-McDermid (PMS) or deletion 22q13 syndrome (OMIM 606232), which is a rare genetic disorder with a highly complex clinical type. PMS genetic defects consist of 22q11.13 deletions or chromosomal structural rearrangements affecting the *SHANK3* gene; lack of *SHANK3* gene function mutations has been reported in a minority of instances. Often there is underdiagnosis of PMS. There are no established clinical diagnostic criteria for PMS and it does not have scientifically defined diagnosis requirements. In this chapter, the researchers identify three cases of PMS and review the clinical and genetic diagnostic methods of this disease, highlighting the function of chromosomal microarray technology in diagnosis of unusual but significant DNA copy number abnormalities

Chapter 7 by Dr. Herrera from the Human Photosynthesis Research Centre in México, describes the unsuspected intrinsic property of melanin to dissociate water molecules, such as chlorophyll in plants, and its implications in the context of chromosomal abnormalities. Chromosome defects, down to the level of the nucleotide, can shed light on the essence of the processes by which normal anatomy forms and abnormal anatomy occurs. It is a daunting challenge to associate genotype with phenotype. Dr. Herrera addresses the energy that guides the development, proper processing, and multiplication of chromosome codes, known as sunlight radiation, through examining melanin.

Chapter 8 "Polyploidy in the ginger family from Thailand," by Dr. Anamthawat-Jónsson from Iceland and Dr. from Umpunjun from Thailand, discusses in detail the taxonomic classification of the ginger family (Zingiberaceae). The ginger family comprises about 50 genera and more than 1300 species worldwide. Approximately 21 genera with about 200 species have been described in Thailand. In this chapter, the researchers include an introduction to Zingiberaceae, which includes the two most cultivated genera, the ginger genus *Zingiber* and the turmeric genus *Curcuma*, and identify their own cytotaxonomic and molecular cytogenetic work on Thailand's *Curcuma* species.

In the final chapter, "Maize chromosome abnormalities and breakage-fusion-bridge cycles in callus cultures," Dr. Aguiar-Perecin et al. from Brazil summarize the maize karyotype, which was first described by the detection of pachytene chromosomes.

The somatic chromosomes with repeated DNA sequences were detected by C-banding and FISH C-banding, which has helped to classify chromosome abnormalities in callus cultures. In this chapter, the authors focus on heterochromatic knobs implicated in the occurrence of chromosome abnormalities in callus cultures. They found anaphase bridges arising from delayed chromatid separation at knob regions and standard bridges in culture originating from dicentric chromatids, and the phenomenon of uneven crossing over in a knob region was observed in callus culture. These results are of interest for studies on the mechanisms of chromosome alterations during evolution.

Tülay Aşkin Çelik
Department of Biology,
Art and Science Faculty,
Aydın Adnan Menderes University,
Aydın, Turkey

Subrata Dey
Maulana Abul Kalam Azad University of Technology
(Formerly West Bengal University of Technology),
Kolkata, West Bengal, India

Section 1

Introduction

Chapter 1

Introductory Chapter: Chromosomal Abnormalities

Tülay Aşkin Çelik

1. Introduction

DNA molecules are tightly wrapped around proteins called histones, non-histone proteins that make structures called **chromosomes,** and are present in the cell nucleus as unconcentrated during the cell cycle. Chromosomes are structures inside cells that contain an individual's genes. The human genomes have 46 chromosomes, composed of 22 pairs of autosomes and a pair of sex chromosomes (X and/or Y). All of the somatic cells in females carry two X chromosomes, and all of the somatic cells in males carry one X and one Y chromosome. One half of each pair of chromosomes comes from through the egg cells; one half of each pair comes from through the sperm cells. As a result, females carry two copies of each X-linked gene, while males carry only one copy of X-linked and Y-linked genes. They vary in size and appearance, the X being much somewhat bigger than the Y and contain entirely separate genes, but they do have small areas of resemblance. Both individuals of a species contain the same number of chromosomes specific for that species. Nonetheless, there are individuals that exhibit differences in this standard complement. Such differences may be changes in number of chromosomes or structural changes inside and within chromosomes, collectively such changes are called chromosomal aberrations or chromosomal anomalies.

Over the past few decades, genetic and genomic advancements have changed our understanding about health. Genetic anomalies are also related to pregnancy and birth defects. Any disease is partly caused by the individual's genetic characteristics. These genetic abnormalities cause genetic defects that arise as a result of changes (mutations) in a person's DNA. Such variations in DNA occur on nucleotide sequences called genes. In this case, the function of the affected gene(s) may be impaired. The disturbance in the structure of the gene will disturb the normal structure and function of proteins. Mutations change the protein coding sequence of the genome in some way. Nonetheless, there are potentially several different pathways that can impair natural gene expression which can lead to genetic defects. Many genes are dominantly transmitted down the family, in which, the individual bears a regular copy and a modified copy of the gene. The altered gene is therefore prevalent or superior to the regular gene. This occurrence triggers a genetic disorder effect to the child. This case is a spontaneous phenomenon. In all boys and girls, this possibility is the same throughout each birth, and the altered gene cannot be reversed and remain constant in one's life. Many dominant or recessive genetic disorders affect the child from birth, while others have an adult effect on the person only. An organism's genetic component regulates its development and its interplay with its environment. Consequently, any change in this genetic material results in variation in phenotypic characters. These effects can vary, depending on the extent of the aberrations, from being lethal to being harmless. Normally, the cell divisions in daughter cells should have an equal number of chromosomes. The duplicated chromosomes must be specifically separated into daughter cells during the cell division. However, too few or too many copies of a chromosome will transfer through daughter cells as a result of cell division errors.

Chromosome abnormalities are mostly the result of a cell division malfunction. A chromosomal abnormality happens when fetus has wrong amount of DNA in a cell; the chromosomes are structurally deficient, or the number of chromosomes is wrong. Additionally, errors can occur in the cell cycle when coping chromosomes. During meiosis division and fertilization, a wide range of chromosomal abnormalities exist; they can be classified into two classes, namely numerical and structural abnormalities. For the gain or loss of a whole chromosome, numerical variations or aneuploidies arise. The resulting phenotypes in a single chromosome or chromosomal fragment are triggered by the mismatch in one or more dosage-sensitive genes. These imbalances in the number of chromosomes also interact with the dose-sensitive and developmentally essential genes and ultimately induce the emergence of unique and complex phenotypes [1, 2]. As a consequence, numerical chromosomal aberrations may be symptomatic of tension on DNA replication without actual chromosome segregation defects. Although most human chromosomal DNA dose not encode proteins, even rather small pieces of chromosomes that contain hundreds of genes [3, 4].

A mutation in a chromosome is an unpredictable change. Quite commonly such modifications are caused by complications that arise during meiosis, or by mutagens such as toxins, radiation, viruses, etc. Chromosome mutations may result in changes in cell count or changes in chromosome structure. Mutations in the composition of chromosomes are variations that affect whole chromosomes and whole genomes rather than just individual nucleotides. Chromosome mutations can cause a large variety of genetic disorders. Chromosome abnormalities are also the cause of early pregnancy loss, fetal malformations, stillbirth, and male infertility associated with it. Addition or deletion of entire chromosomes (aneuploidy) will also have fatal consequences. Aneuploid cells exhibits particular defects in the cell cycle kinetics, growth rate, metabolism, and response to specific stresses [3, 5]. Chromosomal disorders may lead to mental retardation or other developmental problems. For more than one system, phenotypic results of a certain gene typically provide details on the biological roles of the particular gene. Furthermore, a deletion or replication of a single gene that may cause other genes affecting several phenotypes are considered pleiotropic genes [2, 6]. Pleiotropy indicates that certain proteins have more than one role in various types of cells, and any genetic alteration that change the gene expression or function of different tissues will theoretically have far-reaching consequences [6, 7].

Contrary to numeric abnormalities, structural chromosomal abnormalities result from a break or breaks that disrupt the continuity of a chromosome. Sometimes a spontaneous break or breaks occur in a chromosome or chromosomes in a different cell which may lead to deletion, inversion, translocation, isochromosome, and ring chromosome [8]. During the cell division, a part of chromosome content is destroyed; the intrinsic rearrangement becomes unbalanced [9]. A disease may arise as a result of a balanced rearrangement if the breaks in the chromosomes occur in a gene, resulting in a missing or nonfunctional protein, or if the fusion of chromosomal segments results in a two gene combination, creating a new protein product whose work damages the cell. Some of the developmental abnormalities found in embryos are closely linked to chromosomal defects that occur, such as mosaism, haploidy, and polyploidy [10–13].

The classical and molecular cytogenetic techniques provide significant potential applications, especially in clinical trials and biomedical diagnosis, rendering them a strong to other molecular and genomic methods and chromosomal abnormalities.

Genetic knowledge can influence not just the entire populations, but the generations come too. Medical genetics' primary aim is to help individuals with a genetic disorder, their families to lead a life as normal as possible, and to provide adequate care or social support systems.

Biochemical genetics and cytogenetics work in numerous research fields, such as induce genes defects, chromosome-specific zone recognition, and molecular mechanism of chromosomal abnormalities. The advances in genetic testing using molecular biotechnology and mass screening systems for newborn infants help to understand the role of genes, their behavior, the interaction between genetic diseases and environment, the causes of their appearance, and the development of successful therapies and technologies.

Author details

Tülay Aşkin Çelik
Department of Biology, Art and Science Faculty, Aydin Adnan Menderes University, Central Campus, Aydin, Turkey

*Address all correspondence to: tcelik@adu.edu.tr

References

[1] Hassold T, Chen N, Funkhouser J, Jooss T, Manuel B, et al. A cytogenetic study of 1000 spontaneous abortions. Annals of Human Genetics. 1980;**44**(2):151-178

[2] Theisen A, Shaffer LG. Disorders caused by chromosome abnormalities. The Application of Clinical Genetics. 2010;**3**:159-174

[3] Skvorak Giersch AB, Morton CC. Cytogenetics and cochlear expressed sequence tags (ests) for identification of genes involved in hearing and deafness. In: Keats BJB, Fay RR, Popper AN, editors. Genetics of Auditory Disorders. Springer Handbook of Auditory Research. Vol. 14. New York, NY: Springer; 2002. pp. 92-120

[4] Sansregret L, Vanhaesebroeck B, Swanton C. Determinants and clinical implications of chromosomal instability in cancer. Nature Reviews. Clinical Oncology. 2018;**15**(3):139-150

[5] Malumbres M. Control of the cell cycle. Chapter 4. In: Niederhuber et al., editors. Abeloff's Clinical Oncology. 6th ed. Elsevier; 2014. pp. 52-68

[6] Lobo I. Pleiotropy: One gene can affect multiple traits. Nature Education. 2008;**1**(1):10

[7] Wagner A. The role of population size, pleiotropy and fitness effects of mutations in the evolution of overlapping gene functions. Genetics. 2000;**154**(3):1389-1401

[8] Mitelman F, Johansson B, Mertens F. The impact of translocations and gene fusions on cancer causation. Nature Reviews. Cancer. 2007;7(4):233-245

[9] Skvorak Giersch AB. Congenital cytogenetic abnormalities. In: Milunsky A, editor. Genetic Disorders and the Fetus: Diagnosis, Prevention and Treatment. 5th ed. Vol. 1. Baltimore: The Johns Hopkins University Press; 2004. p. 224

[10] Kloosterman WP, Guryev V, van Roosmalen M, Duran KJ, de Bruijin E, et al. Chromothripsis as a mechanism driving complex de novo structural rearrangements in the germline. Human Molecular Genetics. 2011;**20**(10):1916-1924

[11] Liu P, Erez A, Sreenath Nagamani SC, Dhar SU, Kołodziejska KE, Dharmadhikari AV, et al. Chromosome catastrophes involve replication mechanisms generating complex genomic rearrangements. Cell. 2011;**146**(6):889-903

[12] Chiang C, Jacobsen JC, Ersnt C, Hanscom C, Heilbut A, Bluementhal I, et al. Complex reorganization and predominant non-homologous repair following chromosomal breakage in karyotypically balanced germline rearrangements and transgenic integration. Nature Genetics. 2012;**44**(4):390-397

[13] Kloosterman WP, Tavakoli-Yaraki M, van Roosmalen MJ, van Binsbrgen E, Renkens I, et al. Constitutional chromothripsis rearrangements involve clustered double-stranded DNA breaks and nonhomologous repair mechanisms. Cell Reports. 2012;**1**(6):648-655

Section 2

Chromosomal Abnomalities Observed in Humans

Chapter 2

The Risk of Chromosomal Abnormalities in Cases of Minor and Major Fetal Anomalies in the Second Trimester

Artúr Beke and Aténé Simonyi

Abstract

Currently, noninvasive intrauterine screening for most chromosome abnormalities is available, but ultrasound examinations also play an important role during pregnancy, by drawing the attention to the suspect of a possible abnormality. Fetal ultrasound disorders can be classified into two major groups: (1) Major abnormalities are actually diagnosed malformations that are often associated with certain chromosome abnormalities but may be associated with other disorders (multiplex malformation) and may occur as isolated disorders (e.g., cardiac disorders, duodenal atresia, omphalocele, cystic hygroma (CH)). (2) Minor anomalies ("soft markers") are not abnormal in themselves but are mild abnormalities that may occur in normal pregnancy but also increase the risk of certain chromosome aberrations. The minor anomalies in the second trimester include thickened nuchal fold (NF), mild ventriculomegaly, pyelectasis, hyperechogenic bowels, hyperechogenic papillary muscle, and shorter long bones. Plexus choroid cyst which is classified as a minor marker does not increase the risk of Down syndrome but increases the risk of trisomy 18 (Edwards syndrome). We want to emphasize the importance of screening of minor and major ultrasound abnormalities in detecting chromosomal abnormalities in the second trimester.

Keywords: obstetric genetics, prenatal diagnosis, chromosomal abnormalities, prenatal ultrasound, fetal anomalies

1. Introduction

The chromosomal abnormalities account for a considerable part of the anomalies of the intrauterine fetus. Chromosomal abnormalities are the numerical (aneuploidies) and structural anomalies, which can be demonstrated by special methods of examination. The numerical and structural anomalies can be duplications/trisomies, deletions/monosomies, and other rearrangements on the chromosomes.

The autosomal trisomies and unbalanced rearrangements might cause severe multiple malformation syndromes and mental retardation. The rate of the intrauterine deaths is high. They cause mainly severe diseases; in some cases they are associated with anomalies which are incompatible with the postnatal life.

Besides the age, a history of aneuploidy, and noninvasive tests, positive ultrasound findings—which could be major structural abnormalities or minor ultrasound markers—can be an indicator for chromosome analysis [1].

2. Abnormalities with subcutaneous edema

As the first-trimester nuchal edemas (nuchal translucency, NT), the second-trimester nuchal edemas (nuchal thickening, nuchal fold, NF) also elevate the risk of chromosome abnormalities. It is important to distinguish nuchal edema and cystic hygroma (CH), and in the case of nonimmune hydrops (NH), it is also important to discuss cases with or without cystic hygroma separately.

Abnormalities with subcutaneous edema (nonimmune hydrops (NH), cystic hygroma, nuchal edema) increase the risk of chromosome abnormalities. They may warn of a possible intrauterine infection; in the case of nonimmune hydrops, for example, parvovirus B19 infection may occur. They may also be indicative of other pathologies accompanied with fetal anemia, including thalassemia, twin-to-twin transfusion, and disorders of fetal circulation and abnormal anatomy of the fetal heart.

2.1 Nuchal fold (nuchal thickening) in the second trimester

In the second trimester, we examine the thickened nuchal fold (nuchal thickening, NF) in the horizontal section, level with the cerebellum and also containing the cavum septum pellucidum and the cisterna magna. This method, in contrast to the one used in the first trimester, measures the thickness of the soft tissue from the external aspect of the skin to the external aspect of the bone. Authors suggest 5 mm as a cutoff value [2, 3]. A large nuchal translucency detected in the first trimester is a non-specific malformation, and in most cases it resolves during the second trimester of the pregnancy, although it might persist in certain cases to show a picture of nuchal thickening. It indicates an increased risk of trisomy 21 (Down syndrome) [4].

Benacerraf et al. were the first in drawing the attention to the fact that the nuchal fold or nuchal thickening (≥6 mm) observed during the ultrasound examination in the second trimester increases the risk of Down syndrome [4].

Numerous authors carried out similar examinations, subsequently demonstrating different results. Gray and Crane [3] tried to determine the proper cutoff values of nuchal thickening. They formulated two groups according to the size of the pregnancy, putting the values measured in weeks 14–18 to the first group and the data of weeks 19–24 to the second group. Considering the examinations, the suggested cutoff value in the first group (weeks 14–18) is ≥5 mm, and in the second group (weeks 19–24), it is ≥6 mm [5]. In their investigations, Gray and Crane [3] detected pathological karyotypes in 12 out of 47 cases (25.53%). Analyzing 23 cases, DeVore and Alfi found pathological karyotypes in 9 cases (39.13%) [6].

Other authors detected pathological karyotypes in 10% of second-trimester nuchal edema. Grandjean and Sarramon [7] processed the data of 3308 ultrasound examinations, with the help of 12 centers, and they found nuchal thickening in 38% of the cases of trisomy 21. According to the records of 12 centers, they performed karyotyping of 295 pregnancies in the second trimester with nuchal thickening. They found abnormal chromosomes in 22 cases (7.46%), 17 of these were trisomy 21 (5.76%) [7]. Gonen et al. [8] carried out karyotyping in 573 cases because of positive ultrasound findings during ultrasound examinations in the second trimester. There were 38 chromosome analyses carried out due to nuchal thickenings; in one case they found an abnormal karyotype (2.63%) [8]. Zimmer et al. discussed their cases of early second-trimester nuchal edema in 43 out of 1254 cases (3.43%); they detected pathological karyotypes, trisomy 21 being the chief cause in 27 cases, while other pathological karyotypes were blamed in 16 cases [9].

Beke et al. [10] showed a value within 10% in the case of nuchal fold (thickening) measured in the second trimester. A total of 254 cases of chromosomal examination was performed for second-trimester nuchal edema, and in 14 cases, an abnormal karyotype was detected (5.51%). With the highest frequency, monosomy X occurred (nine cases, 3.54%), while in three cases trisomy 21, in 1-1 cases trisomy 18 (Edwards syndrome), and another chromosome abnormality were detected [10].

2.2 Cystic hygroma

Cystic hygroma is observable in the first and second trimesters. It can be differentiated from nuchal translucency and nuchal thickening by the clearly isolated fluid space and the typical medial line septation shown on ultrasound examination [11, 12]. Cystic hygroma often persists and is often associated with aneuploidy (mainly monosomy X), other abnormalities, and fetal loss [12].

In the case of cystic hygroma, the risk of the chromosome abnormality is even higher than in cases of nuchal thickening. Bronshtein et al. found chromosome anomalies in 6 of 106 nonseptated cases (5.66%), whereas the risk of the chromosome abnormality in the 25 septated cases was 72% [12].

Nadel et al. [13] examined in separate groups those cases where the cystic hygroma occurred by itself (isolated) and those where it was a part of the hydrops phenomenon. In cases of individually occurring 26 hygromas, there were chromosome abnormalities in 12 cases (46.15%), while in hydrops-associated cases (37 cases), they found 31 chromosome anomalies (83.78%) [13]. Due to cystic hygroma, Gonen et al. detected 15 cases of pathological (abnormal) karyotype in 182 cases (8.24%) [8]. Sohn and Gast [14] found 20 cases of abnormal karyotype of the 57 cystic hygroma cases (35.09%). There were 11 cases of monosomy X (Turner syndrome), 5 cases of trisomy 21, and 4 cases of trisomy 18 [14]. Taipale et al. carried out karyotyping in 76 cases of cystic hygroma, and they found chromosome abnormalities in 18 cases (23.68%), monosomy X in 5 cases, trisomy 21 in 7 cases, and trisomy 13 (Patau syndrome) and trisomy 18 in 6 cases [15].

Beke et al. [10] had a similar result. In terms of isolated cystic hygroma, fetal chromosome examinations were performed in 27 cases, and in 13 cases abnormal karyotypes were detected (48.15%). When cystic hygroma was associated with hydrops, a total of 13 cases was investigated, and 7 cases of chromosomal abnormalities (53.85%) were detected [10].

In the first and early second trimesters, Rosati and Guariglia [16] examined the volume of cystic hygromas by volumetric calculations. They also analyzed the proportion of associated chromosomal abnormalities, and in 8 of 14 septated cases, they detected pathological karyotypes (57.14%), whereas four pathological karyotypes (21.05%) were seen in the 19 nonseptated cases. In summary, the 12 patients with chromosomal abnormalities (36.36%) were divided as follows: trisomy 21 in 6 patients, monosomy X in 4 cases, and trisomy 18 and 13 in 1 case each [16]. Examining the septated and nonseptated cases together, Tanriverdi et al. found 13 pathological karyotypes (56.52%) among the 23 karyotyped patients [17]. Donnenfeld et al. applied karyotyping and fluorescent in situ hybridization (FISH) in the chromosomal investigation of the cells in the sample obtained from the fluid of the cystic hygroma and could justify monosomy X in 86% [18].

Examining a total of 218 fetuses with subcutaneous edema, Gezer et al. [19] found that nuchal fold, cystic hygroma, and nonimmune hydrops could be significant markers for abnormal chromosome numbers. Of these 218 cases, 71 (32.57%) were diagnosed with abnormal karyotype. The percentage breakdown in 71 cases was as follows: 37% monosomy X, 44% trisomy 21, 15% trisomy 18, and 4% trisomy 13 [19].

2.3 Nonimmune hydrops

Similarly to cystic hygroma, nonimmune hydrops can be observed both in the first and second trimesters and is often associated with aneuploidy (monosomy X or trisomy 21) and fetal loss [13].

Nicolaides et al. studied 37 cases in 1986 and demonstrated 12 cases of chromosome anomalies (32.43%) [20]. Gembruch et al. found 17 abnormal karyotypes examining 45 hydrops cases (37.78%), 10 cases of monosomy X (1 mosaic form), 6 cases of trisomy 21, and 1 case of trisomy 18 [21].

Boyd and Keeling [22] and Anandakumar et al. [23] found X-monosomies in 50% of the demonstrated chromosome abnormalities. Boyd and Keeling [22] found 11 X-monosomies of the 22 cases of chromosome anomalies of the 72 nonimmune hydrops cases (30.56%), while Anandakumar et al. [23] carried out karyotyping in cases of 100 hydrops-affected fetuses and demonstrated 5 cases of X-monosomies of 10 abnormal cases (10%).

Schwanitz et al. examined in separate groups the nonimmune hydrops cases associated with cystic hygroma and the individually occurring ones. When it was associated with cystic hygroma, abnormal karyotypes were demonstrated in 54.39%; without cystic hygroma this rate was 27.69% [24].

Has carried out investigations into nonimmune hydrops in the first trimester and found 9 pathological karyotypes (47.37%) out of 19 cases [25].

In the case of nonimmune hydrops, Beke et al. found chromosomal abnormalities in 4 out of 20 cases (20%), in each case monosomy X [10].

3. Cerebral and cranial anomalies

In the case of ventriculomegaly, a greater than normal amount of liquor expands the ventricular system. Cerebrospinal fluid may be overproduced, impaired, or obstructed. Increased pressure leads to thinning of the brain, creating hydrocephalus internus. Hydrocephalus externus is referred to as the proliferation of liquor in the subarachnoid space. Ultrasound first shows the expansion of the posterior horn of the side chamber. In cases of choroid plexus cyst and other cranial malformations, the risk of chromosomal abnormalities is also elevated.

3.1 Ventriculomegaly

In cases of cerebral anomalies, we define ventricular dilatation (ventriculomegaly) as a lateral ventricle with a diameter $\geq$ 10 mm. The ventricle of normal male fetuses is mildly wider (average 6.4 mm) than of the ventricle of normal female fetuses (average 5.8 mm) [26]. Ventriculomegaly increases the incidence rate of aneuploidy (trisomy 21 and other aneuploidies) [27, 28].

Several authors were examining ventriculomegaly as one possible marker of the fetal chromosome abnormalities in the second trimester. Nicolaides et al. carried out karyotyping in 9 cases because of fetal ventriculomegaly, examining this among other anomalies, and they found chromosome abnormalities in 2 cases (22.22%) [20]. Following this, Mahony et al. [28] found 1 case of 20 ventriculomegalies (5%); Bromley et al. [27] observed 5 cases of chromosome anomalies examining 44 cases of ventriculomegaly (11.36%). The study of Gonen et al. [8] also extended to more anomalies; as a part of it, they carried out karyotyping in 25 cases of ventriculomegalies and found no abnormal karyotypes. Terry et al. [29] detected abnormal chromosomes in 3 cases of the 25 examined fetuses (12%).

Beke et al. [30] found different karyotypes in 26 (6.25%) out of the 416 examined fetuses. If ventriculomegaly was isolated (191 cases), the rate of the chromosome abnormality was 3.7% (7 cases). In four cases, trisomy 21 was detected, in two cases monosomy X, and in one case trisomy 18. Lateral ventricular dilation (ventriculomegaly) was associated with other ultrasound findings in 225 cases, and in 19 of these, there were chromosome abnormalities detected (8.4%). The distribution of pathological (abnormal) karyotypes was as follows: 4-4 cases of monosomy X and 47, XXY karyotype (Klinefelter syndrome), 3-3 cases of trisomy 21 and trisomy 18, and 1-1 case of trisomy 13, 47,XXX, 47,XYY, 49,XXXY karyotypes and triploidy were detected. We found a higher rate in cases of bilateral anomaly (ventriculomegaly) (8.6%) than in unilateral cases (4.6%) [30].

3.2 Choroid plexus cysts

According to the data of more authors, the choroid plexus cysts (CPC) mainly increase the risk for trisomy 18 [31, 32]. According to certain studies, the risk level does not depend on whether the anomaly is unilateral or bilateral, but other studies show that the larger the anomaly (>10 mm), the higher the risk [33, 34]. Certain authors suggest the 2–2.5 mm cutoff value [35], while others determined the 5 mm limiting value [33]. The cysts resolve practically every time, so the absence of the anomaly on a repeated ultrasound examination does not indicate a decrease in the risk [36].

Chudleigh et al. were the first who described cysts in the fetal choroid plexus [37]. Nicolaides et al. were the first who drew attention to the connection between the positive ultrasound finding of choroid plexus cysts and chromosome abnormalities, through a study including a small number of cases [20]. Thereafter, more authors demonstrated that fetal choroid plexus cysts mainly increase the risk of trisomy 18 and, to a lesser degree, the risk of trisomy 21.

Achiron et al. demonstrated 2 trisomy 18 cases from chromosome analysis of 30 CPC cases (6.67%); in 1 case the CPC was associated with other ultrasound anomalies [38]. Platt et al. found 4 cases of chromosome abnormalities from 62 cases (6.45%), in 3 cases it was trisomy 18, and in 1 case it was trisomy 21 [39]. Nadel et al. demonstrated 12 cases (5.13%) of abnormal chromosomes from a larger number of cases (234 cases), 11 of which were trisomy 18 (4.7%) and 1 case of triploidy, but from 234 cases there were 220 cases of isolated CPC, and in these cases they did not detect any chromosome abnormalities [40].

Walkinshaw et al. demonstrated 4 cases (2.63%) of chromosome anomalies out of 152 isolated CPC cases, 3 cases trisomy 18 (1.97%) and 1 case trisomy 21 [33]. Nava et al. found eight chromosome abnormalities in 176 cases (4.55%), 4 cases of trisomy 18 (2.27%), 2 cases of trisomy 21 (1.14%), 1 case of 47, XXY karyotype, and 1 case of another chromosome anomaly [41]. From the trisomy 18 cases, there was one case of isolated choroid plexus cyst, while in three cases the abnormality was associated with other ultrasound findings. Gonen et al. in 1995 demonstrated no abnormalities in the course of intrauterine karyotyping of 108 CPC cases [8].

Gray et al. performed karyotyping in 208 cases, and they detected abnormal karyotypes in 7 cases; each case was trisomy 18 (3.37%) [34]. Bakos et al. found 3 abnormal karyotypes out of 108 examined cases (2.78), 1 case was trisomy 18, and 1 case was trisomy 13 and one inversion of chromosome 9 [42].

Chitty et al. [43] with a larger number of cases found chromosome abnormalities in 14 cases (2.13%). They examined separately the isolated cases and the cases associated with other ultrasound anomalies. In 603 cases, the choroid plexus cyst was not associated with other ultrasound abnormalities, and in 3 cases (0.5%), they found abnormal karyotypes (each was trisomy 18); in 55 cases the abnormality was associated with other ultrasound findings, and in 11 cases (20%), they detected abnormal karyotypes (in 9 cases trisomy 18, in one case trisomy 21, and in 1 case 47,XXX karyotype) [43]. With a similarly large number of cases, Ghidini et al. examined the incidence of chromosome abnormalities in cases of choroid plexus cysts, they only examined the isolated cases (765 cases), and they found abnormal karyotypes (trisomy 18) in 13 cases (1.7%) [44].

Coco et al. [45] in 2004 examined separately the isolated cases and those associated with other abnormalities, the cases associated with minor and major ultrasound anomalies. The rate of abnormal karyotypes was 0.55% in total. In isolated cases (311 cases) and in associated cases with minor anomalies (43 cases), they did not find any abnormal karyotypes. In the two detected cases of trisomy 18, the choroid plexus cyst was associated with major anomalies (16.67% from 12 cases) [45]. Sahinoglu et al. [46] performed karyotyping in 109 cases due to choroid plexus cyst, 3.67% of the patients had an abnormal karyotype, in 102 cases, it was isolated anomaly, and in 3 cases they found chromosome abnormalities (2.94%). In seven cases, the choroid plexus cysts were associated with other ultrasound anomalies, and they found chromosome abnormality in one case (14.29%); in all the detected four cases, the abnormal karyotype was trisomy 18.

According to a 2008 study, of the 435 cases identified by CPC, 390 undertook karyotyping. Of these, anomalies were found in 14 fetuses (3.59%), with the highest frequency being trisomy 18 (6 cases, 1.54%); in 1 case trisomy 21 (1, 0.26%) and 1 case trisomy 9 (0.26%) were detected. The incidence of monosomy X was 0.77% (3 cases). In one case, 47, XXY karyotype (0.26%) and in two cases other chromosomal abnormalities (0.51%) were confirmed (46,XX/46,XY and 46,XY/47,XXY/47,XYY mosaicism). Of the cases studied, other ultrasound abnormalities associated with the plexus cyst were found in 178 pregnancies, and 7 abnormal karyotypes were found (3.93%), 5 cases of trisomy 18, and 2 cases of monosomy X. Choroid plexus cyst occurred as an isolated anomaly in 212 pregnancies (it was not associated with any other fetal ultrasound findings (anomalies) and/or poly/oligohydramnios), and 7 chromosome abnormalities (3.3%) were found, one of which was trisomy 18, 1 case trisomy 21, 1 case trisomy 9, 1 case monosomy X, and 1 case 47,XXY karyotype. The incidence of chromosome abnormalities was also similar in the case of unilateral and bilateral CPC; chromosome abnormalities were detected in the case of unilateral (3.3%) and in the case of bilateral anomalies (3.9%) [47].

3.3 Other cranial and cerebral anomalies

Other cranial and cerebral anomalies (holoprosencephaly, agenesis or dysgenesis of the corpus callosum, Dandy-Walker malformation, and cleft lip or palate) according to observations increase the risk of chromosome abnormalities, but they do not increase the risk of trisomy 21 [48]. A strawberry-shaped head mainly increases the risk of trisomy 18 [49].

Benacerraf et al. reported five cases already in 1984, where they found intrauterine cleft lip and palate and holoprosencephaly during the ultrasound examinations, and the chromosome analysis verified trisomy 13 in two cases (33.33%) [50].

Both Parant et al. [51] and later Tongsong et al. [52] reported 12 cases where they diagnosed intrauterine holoprosencephaly. The karyotyping in Parant et al. [51]'s study verified trisomy 13 in four cases (33.33%); in Tongsong et al. [52]'s study, there were three cases of trisomies found (25%); in two cases it was trisomy 13 (16.67%), and in one case it was trisomy 18 (8.33%). Bullen et al. reported in their study (2001) 68 cases of holoprosencephaly, they made karyotyping in 52 cases, where they found an abnormal karyotype in 38% (from 20 cases in 15 cases it was trisomy 13, in 2 cases trisomy 18, and in 3 cases other chromosome anomalies, from which in 2 cases they recognized the deletion of the long arm of chromosome 13) [53]. Studying the etiology of the holoprosencephaly, besides the maternal diabetes and trisomy 13, there are also monogenic types [54].

In cases of cleft lip and/or palate, Perrotin et al. [55] demonstrated in their study that in those cases they examined, there were no chromosome anomalies provided the abnormality was isolated (14 cases), and when they detected it together with other positive ultrasound findings, the incidence rate of the chromosome abnormalities was high. In 26 cases, there were 15 chromosome anomalies (57.69%), in 8 cases trisomy 13, and in 5 cases trisomy 18 [55].

Aletebi and Fung [56] studied the abnormalities of the fossa posterior region, including the enlarged cisterna magna, the Dandy-Walker malformation, and the fossa posterior cyst. They found chromosome abnormalities (trisomy 18) in 1 of 15 cases (6.67%) [56].

Similarly, Beke et al. found in their study that the frequency of chromosome abnormalities was similar to other cranial abnormalities; with 44 fetuses being examined, they detected chromosome abnormalities in 7 cases (15.91%) [30].

The aim of Nazer Herrera et al. [57] was to estimate the prevalence of holoprosencephaly in relation to births. It turned out that this disorder occurred with low frequency in Chile, but it was associated with a high proportion of trisomy 13: occurring in 10.91% of the cases examined (6 out of 55 cases) [57].

In another study, this anatomical disorder and chromosome abnormalities were associated with a high proportion. According to a study in Japan, five out of seven holoprosencephaly cases (71.43%) showed the following differences: two children with trisomy 18, two children with trisomy 13, and one with 45,X karyotype [58].

4. Cardiac and thoracic abnormalities

The use of fetal echocardiography may further increase the importance of second-trimester ultrasound examinations for screening for chromosomal anomalies. This is particularly true in those cases where screening tests were not available in the first trimester or the pregnancy was only recognized later.

4.1 Echogenic intracardiac focus

In the fetal heart, the echogenic intracardiac focus is observable in 3–4% of normal pregnancies [59]; according to some studies, this rate might reach 10% in the Asian population [60]. Its incidence, by some authors, increases the risk of trisomy 21 [61–65] and, according to some studies, trisomy 13 [66]. According to some literature data, the risk is higher if the anomaly is observable in both ventricles [61].

Bromley et al. [61, 62] examined in their studies (reported in 1995 and 1998) the correlation between the chromosome anomalies and the echogenic intracardiac focus detected during the ultrasound examinations. In 1995 they studied 66 cases and found trisomy 21 in 4 cases (6.06%) [61]. Chromosome abnormalities were found in 14 cases (4.83%) with a higher number of cases (290). In 1998, they examined 290 pregnancies in two groups and detected chromosome abnormalities (mainly trisomy 21) in 6.4% (125 cases) in that group where the maternal age was ≥35 years, and in the age group under 35 years (165 cases), this rate was 3.64% [62]. Winter et al. demonstrated in their similar report 16 cases of trisomy 21 of the studied 163 cases (9.28%) [65].

In a 2005 publication, the echogenic papillary muscle showed abnormal karyotype only when it was associated with other anomalies (4.69%), not in isolated cases [30].

4.2 Ventricular septal defect and atrioventricular septal defect

Many authors investigated the correlation among the chromosome abnormalities and the ventricular septal defect (VSD) and the atrioventricular septal defect (AVSD). In some cases, the authors managed the cases discovered in the second trimester or later in pregnancy (third trimester) and the cases diagnosed after birth as aggregated data. Hajdu et al. studied 21 cases of AVSD and found chromosome anomalies in 9 cases (42.86%); 7 of these were trisomy 21, 1 case trisomy 18, and 1 case trisomy 22 [67].

Tennstedt et al. [68] analyzed all those cases where the fetopathological examination verified cardiac malformation, and there were ultrasound examinations and karyotyping during the pregnancy (altogether 129 cases). A total of 36 fetuses had VSD, and 21 fetuses had AVSD. In cases of VSD, there were 15 fetuses (41.67%) with detected chromosome anomalies (8 cases of trisomy 21, 4 cases of trisomy 18, 1 case of trisomy 13, 2 cases of other abnormalities). If AVSD occurred, the incidence rate of the chromosome anomalies was 61.9% (from 13 cases, 9 trisomy 21 and 3 trisomy 18, and in 1 case other anomaly) [68]. Delisle et al. [69] studied the incidence of the chromosome abnormalities in cases of AVSD detected by ultrasound examinations during pregnancy, and from the 38 cases, they found 22 (57.89%) with chromosome anomalies (19 cases of trisomy 21, 1 case of trisomy 18, 1 case of trisomy 13, and 1 case of other positive finding). Paladini et al. [70] reported a study about the risk of chromosome abnormalities in cases of all cardiac (heart and large blood vessels) anomalies. In case of ventricular septal defect, the incidence rate of the chromosome anomalies was 45.33% (34 of 75 cases), and in case of atrioventricular septal defect, this rate was 80% (32 of 40 cases) [70]. From the 34 VSD cases, there were 14 cases of trisomy 21 (18.67%), 16 cases of trisomy 18 (21.33%), 2 cases of monosomy X (2.67%), and 2 other anomalies detectable. The distribution of the 32 abnormal karyotypes in case of AVSD was the following: 26 cases of trisomy 21 (65%), 3 cases of trisomy 18 (7.5%), and 3 other anomalies.

In their work, Beke et al. found abnormalities in 4 out of 18 fetuses with VSD (22.22%), including 2 cases of trisomy 18 (11.11%) and 1 case of trisomy 13 (5.56%) as well as 1 case of another anomaly [30].

Hajdu et al. [71] later, in 2005 in the case of AVSD, the frequency of the abnormal karyotypes was 66.67%. They studied 39 cases of AVSD and found chromosome anomalies in 19 cases (66.67%); 19 of these were trisomy 21, 6 cases trisomy 18, and 1 case trisomy 22 [71].

A 2006 study dealt with the VSD-related clinical characteristics of the Moroccan pediatric population, among others. The 44 patients involved in the research were between 2 and 3 years old. Six of them (13.64%) had Down syndrome. VSD patients who were later subjected to surgical correction were more likely to be able to avoid irreversible pulmonary artery hypertension [72].

According to another, Chinese publication, the association of trisomy 21 is also high in the case of complete AVSD (CAVSD). In a group of 35 patients with this type of anatomical deviation, Zhong et al. performed chromosome tests in 15 cases. A total of 13 chromosome abnormalities (86.67%) have been reported, of which 11 patients with Down syndrome have been identified [73].

Relatively few studies deal with long-term follow-up of Fallot tetralogy cases. According to Shuhaiber et al., the prospects can be positive for those who are being treated surgically in the case of the disease. In their study, however, they also refer to the related VSD and the high proportion of trisomy 21 (80.33%, according to their calculations) in their combined occurrence [74].

4.3 Other cardiac and large blood vessel abnormalities

In cases of other cardiac abnormalities and anomalies of the large blood vessels, the risk of chromosome abnormality is increased [75]. Paladini et al. [70] studied the incidence of the chromosome anomalies in cases of other cardiac and large blood vessel malformations. In the case of coarctation of the aorta, the incidence rate of abnormal chromosomes was 48.28%; in the case of double outlet right ventricle, it was 26.32%; in the case of hypoplastic left heart syndrome, it was 13.51%; in the case of truncus arteriosus, it was 33.33%; in the case of Fallot tetralogy, it was 45%; and in the case of atrial septal defect, there were no abnormal karyotypes found [70].

Other researchers also produced statistics for other heart disorders. Chromosome abnormalities were detected in six cases when investigating 33 fetuses [30].

4.4 Isolated hydrothorax

Only a few authors studied the isolated hydrothorax. Nicolaides carried out karyotyping in three cases because of isolated hydrothorax, in connection with an invasive intervention (blood gained by fetoscopy) performed due to other positive ultrasound findings, and found abnormal karyotype in one case [20]. Estoff et al. carried out karyotyping in 11 cases because of isolated hydrothorax, and in 1 case they found an abnormal karyotype (trisomy 21, 9.09%) [76]. In other studies, in two out of six (33.33%) cases, one case of trisomy 18 (16.67%) and one case of monosomy X (16.67%) associations were observed [30].

5. Abnormalities of the abdominal wall and abdomen

In the case of diaphragmatic hernia, abdominal organs appear in the chest due to a discontinuity in the compartment. About 90% of the lesion is on the left. The aperture of the compartment is not traceable; the abdominal organs of the fetus (liver, stomach, and intestines) appear in the chest, which dislocate the mediastinum and the heart. Chest space narrowing may lead to severe lung hypoplasia.

In cases of an omphalocele, organs (typically the intestines, stomach, and liver) protrude through the opening into the umbilical cord; the opening is in the center (median) of the abdominal wall, where the umbilical cord meets the abdomen.

Among the abdominal wall malformations, gastroschisis is a full-thickness defect of the abdominal wall, typically to the right of the umbilical cord, not including it. Through the open abdominal cavity, the small and large intestines protrude; there is no amnioperitoneal membrane covering the exposed organs.

During the ultrasound screening, the "double bubble" is a characteristic sign of duodenal atresia. The two "bubbles" are the distended stomach and dilated proximal duodenum.

Regarding anomalies of the abdominal wall and abdomen, the structural malformations associated with chromosome abnormalities are omphalocele and duodenal atresia. In cases with echogenic bowel—which is a marker and not necessarily abnormal in itself—the risk of trisomy 21 is higher [77–80]. The etiology of echogenic bowel could be other rare abnormalities (cystic fibrosis, atresia) in addition to the more frequent intrauterine infections [81].

5.1 Diaphragmatic hernia

Blancato et al. [82] demonstrated earlier (1992) by in situ hybridization the occurrence of tissue-specific mosaicism in some cases of diaphragmatic hernia. While during lymphocyte culturing there are no detectable anomalies (blood samples via cordocentesis or blood testing of the newborn), in cases of fibroblast samples (genetic amniocentesis and dermal biopsy), 12p isochromosome can be found. Donnenfeld et al. [83] carried out chromosome analysis in 15 cases of diaphragmatic hernia. In all cases they performed lymphocyte culturing (in 14 cases of fetal cordocentesis) in addition to the fibroblast tests. They found chromosome anomalies in seven cases (46.67%), of which there were three cases of trisomy 18, three cases of 12p mosaicism, and one case of other abnormality [83]. From the seven cases of anomalies, there were two with different results of the cells of different origins due to the mosaicism, and the 12p isochromosome was only detectable from the fibroblasts (amniocentesis and dermal biopsy) and not from the lymphocytes gained from the blood. In five cases, the examinations of the lymphocytes and the fibroblasts gave the same results (three cases of trisomy 18, one case of unbalanced translocation, and one case of 12p isochromosome). Huddy et al. studied 35 cases of diaphragmatic hernia, they examined the outcome of the pregnancy and the related abnormalities, and they found chromosome anomalies in 4 cases altogether (11.43%), of which 2 were trisomy 18 [84].

5.2 Omphalocele (exomphalos)

Many authors studied the abdominal malformations and the other anomalies associated with them. According to all data of the literature, the omphalocele (or exomphalos) is associated with chromosome abnormalities in high rates, mainly with trisomy 18, and in smaller proportion with trisomy 13.

Mann et al. in their study of obstetrical events associated with abdominal malformations reported 7 cases of chromosome abnormalities of 19 cases of omphalocele (36.84%) [85]. Rabe et al. processed the results of similar number of ultrasonographic screening during pregnancy, and in 17 omphalocele cases, they have found 6 chromosome anomalies (35.29%) [86]. Nicolaides et al. in 1986 with a smaller number of cases (8 chromosome abnormalities of 12 cases) [20] and later Gilbert and Nicolaides in 1987 with 19 chromosome anomalies of 35 cases demonstrated [87] that the omphalocele detected by ultrasonographic screening increases the risk of chromosome abnormalities.

Many other scientists verified the results of these studies. Nyberg et al. [88] demonstrated chromosome abnormalities in 10 of 26 cases (38.46%), Holzgreve et al. [89] in 5 of 10 cases (50%), Rizzo et al. [90] in 7 of 12 cases (58.33%), and Fogel et al. [91] in 5 of 37 cases. In their recent study with a higher number of cases, Nicolaides et al. detected abnormal karyotypes in 42 of 116 omphalocele cases (36.21%); 32 cases of these were trisomy 18 (27.59%) and in 7 cases trisomy 13 (6.03%) [92]. Snijders et al. [93] found in higher rate abnormal karyotype, mainly trisomy 18, in 12 of 18 cases (66.67%). The following studies demonstrated almost the same results, Dillon and Renwick [94] in 12 of 43 cases (27.91%), Axt et al. [95] in 7 of 26 cases (26.92%), and Rankin et al. [96] in 30 of 98 cases (30.61%), while Stoll et al. [97] have found abnormal karyotypes in 17 cases out of 58 cases (29.31%). The majority of the abnormal karyotypes were trisomy 18. Axt et al. found the risk of chromosome abnormalities four times higher when the liver was placed intracorporeally than when in the extracorporal placement [95]. Barisic et al. [98] processed the data of 19 European centers and described 34 abnormal karyotypes in total for 137 omphalocele cases (24.82%). Most of the chromosomal abnormalities were trisomy 18 (21 cases, 15.33%); they described a lower rate of trisomy 13 (5 cases, 3.65%), one case of trisomy 21 and monosomy X, two cases of triploidy, and four cases of other chromosomal abnormalities. Salihu et al. [99] processed 29 cases, and 3 abnormal karyotypes were detected (10.34%); in all cases the liver was located intracorporeally.

In the study of Beke et al., out of 21 fetuses diagnosed with omphalocele, two cases (9.52%) were associated with different karyotypes, 1 case trisomy 18, and 1 case trisomy 13 [30].

5.3 Gastroschisis

Many investigators studied the gastroschisis cases in parallel with the omphalocele screenings, even though some of the studies were carried out with a smaller number of cases, so the results are not consistent. Rankin et al. found 1 case of chromosome abnormality in 133 gastroschisis cases (trisomy 13, 0.75%) [96]. Barisic et al. [98] also found abnormal karyotypes in 1.89% at a higher number of cases; they described chromosomal abnormalities in 2 out of the total 106 cases, of which 1 was trisomy 21 and the other was trisomy 13.

Other studies with a smaller number of cases did not indicate chromosome abnormalities; Mann et al. [85] studied 10 cases, Nicolaides et al. [20, 92] 3 and 26 cases, Dillon et al. [94] 56 cases, and Axt et al. [95] 18 cases, and they could not detect any abnormal karyotype. Stoll et al. [97] studied 47 cases of gastroschisis, while Salihu et al. [99] described 15 cases; in these cases there were no abnormal karyotypes detected.

Gastroschisis is often associated with other anomalies. Along with polyhydramnios, special attention should be paid to the ultrasound examination of the fetus. This was observed by Ozawa et al. [100] in a study involving the analysis of 52 fetuses. A quarter of them had trisomy (13 cases, 25%), particularly high rates of Edwards syndrome detected in 10 cases, while Patau syndrome in 2 cases and trisomy 21 in 1 case [100].

In contrast, Stoll et al. [101] diagnosed only one fetus with chromosome abnormality in the case of gastroschisis (trisomy 21) representing 1.16% of the patients studied. They also stated that the etiology of omphalocele and gastroschisis is unclear and their pathogenesis is controversial [101].

5.4 Duodenal atresia (duodenal obstruction)

The ultrasonographic mark of the duodenal obstruction is the "double bubble." The disease is not always detected intrauterine; therefore some investigators involved the subsequently proven, postnatal cases to their study. Studies demonstrated that it mainly increases the risk of trisomy 21. Nicolaides et al. studied 23 cases and found chromosome abnormalities in 10 cases (43.48%) [92]. Bailey et al. detected 15 cases of chromosome anomalies of the 138 cases (trisomy 21) (10.87%) [102]. This rate at Heydanus et al. was 7 abnormal karyotypes out of 29 cases (24.14%), 6 of which were trisomy 21 [103]. Lawrence et al. found 11 cases of chromosome anomalies of also 29 cases (37.93%), in 8 cases trisomy 21 [104]. Beke et al. found abnormalities in 2 out of 17 studied cases (11.76%), including a trisomy 21 [30].

5.5 Echogenic bowel

It is controversial in international literature whether the karyotyping is justified in cases of echogenic bowel. Nyberg et al. was the first to draw the attention to the echogenic bowel increasing mainly the risk of trisomy 21 [105]. Subsequently Scioscia et al. reported 6 cases of chromosome abnormalities of 22 chromosome analyses associated with echogenic bowel (27.27%); in 5 cases trisomy 21 and in 1 case trisomy 18 were found [79]. Bromley et al. carried out 50 karyotyping associated with echogenic bowel and detected abnormal chromosomes in eight cases (16%), six cases of trisomy 21, one case of trisomy 13, and one case of monosomy X [77]. Sipes et al. studied seven cases and detected one case (14.3%) of trisomy 18 [81].

There were two greater studies fully investigating the expectable risk in association with echogenic bowel.

Slotnick and Abuhamad [106] separately screened the different measures of echogenity in their study published in Lancet, classifying them this way: grade1, mild increase of echogenity; grade2, moderate increase; and grade3, pronounced increase. They carried out altogether 145 karyotyping because of echogenic bowel and found abnormal karyotypes (all trisomy 21) in eight cases (5.5%). There were 6 cases of trisomy 21 of the 24 grade3 cases (25%), 2 positive cases of the 81 grade2 cases (2.47%), and no chromosome abnormalities of the 40 cases of grade1. They also studied the incidence of cystic fibrosis, they found 5 cases at grade3 and 2 cases at grade2, and they did not detect any cystic fibrosis at grade1 [106].

Strocker et al. [80] studied those cases separately, where the increasing bowel echogenity was associated with other malformations. They detected abnormal karyotypes in 15 cases of altogether 131 cases (11.45%). In 62 cases, the echogenic bowel was not associated with other positive ultrasonographic findings; in this group, there were 5 chromosome anomalies found, in 4 cases trisomy 21 (6.45%) and 47, XXY karyotype in 1 case. In the other group, there were 69 cases associated with other ultrasonographic findings; 10 of these cases carried chromosome abnormalities, 8 cases trisomy 21 (11.59), 1 case triploidy, and 1 case deletion X [80].

According to the observation of Beke et al., chromosome abnormalities were detected in only 3 out of 53 cases (5.66%), when the ultrasound image of the echogenic bowel was not isolated but associated with other defects [30].

5.6 Other abdominal malformations

Nicolaides et al. [92] also examined other abdominal malformations. In his study there were 24 cases of karyotyping due to lack of a visible stomach, and he found an abnormal karyotype in 18 cases (75%). In other 24 cases of chromosome analyses due to intestinal dilatation, there was 1 with abnormality (4.17%) [92].

6. Pyelectasis

Pyelectasis is the dilatation of only the renal pelvis and the calyces, in milder cases, while when the parenchyma is also affected by the longer lasting compression (becoming thinner), hydronephrosis develops. Obstructions of the urinary tract usually result in the dilatation of the proximal sections. Obstruction of the uretero-pelvic junction is the main cause of hydronephrosis in the neonates.

According to some authors, an increase in the size of the renal pelvis elevates the risk of aneuploidies (mainly trisomy 21) [107–110]. We measure the renal pelvis in a horizontal section in the anteroposterior (AP) direction. We define renal pelvis dilatation (pyelectasis) as a pelvis with an AP dimension ≥5 mm. Hydronephrosis (a renal pelvis ≥10 mm) and enlarged, echogenic kidneys increase the risk of trisomy 13.

Benacerraf et al. [107] studied 210 cases of fetuses with pyelectasis. They found trisomy 21 in 7 of the 210 cases (3.33%). The suggested criteria for pyelectasis were the following cutoff values, ≥4 mm until week 20 and ≥5 mm in weeks 21–30, and after week 30 the limit should be ≥7 mm [107]. Corteville et al. studied 127 cases and detected chromosome abnormalities in 7 cases (5.51%), 4 of these were trisomy 21 (3.15%) [109]. They suggested that until week 33 the cutoff value should be ≥4 mm; after week 33 this limit would be ≥7 mm. Under comparable conditions (121 cases, similar cutoff values), Wickstrom et al. found chromosome anomalies in three cases (2.48%), two of which were trisomy 21 (1.65%) [111].

Nicolaides et al. reported in their study 35 abnormal karyotypes that are found in cases of 258 fetuses with pyelectasis (13.57%) [92]. Their recommended cutoff value was ≥5 mm as a criteria for pyelectasis. Chudleigh et al. carried out chromosome analysis using 5 mm cutoff value in 737 cases of fetal pyelectasis. Studying the results of the karyotyping, they found abnormal chromosomes in 12 cases (1.63%), and 6 of these were trisomy 21 (0.81%) [108]. Besides less number of cases, other scientists did not verify the higher rate of chromosome anomalies. Gonen et al. found no abnormal karyotypes in 58 cases of fetal pyelectasis [8].

Beke et al. [30] processed 302 cases, of which 7 (2.32%) were found to have abnormalities. Of these, 1-1 cases of trisomy 21 and trisomy 18, two cases of monosomy X, and three cases of other chromosome abnormalities were found [30].

According to the findings of a 2006 study, contrary to previous opinions that male fetuses had a higher rate of chromosome abnormalities associated with pyelectasis, they refuted this. According to this new article by Bronstein et al. [112], there is no significant difference between the sexes in the karyotype associated with the anatomical disorder. When investigating 672 cases, 35 (5.21%) cases of abnormal karyotype occurred [112].

Based on Coco's and Jeanty [113]'s findings, pyelectasis alone does not justify an amniocentesis if it is not associated with anatomical and other abnormalities. However, 3.01% of their cases were associated with chromosome abnormalities as well [113].

7. Abnormalities of the extremities

Measuring the length of fetal femur and more recently the humerus is part of the biometric test. Following the limbs of the fetus, the joints, the hands, and the feet and their deviations can be brought into the field of vision. Limb disorders may appear independently or as part of syndromes, causing extensive ossification anomalies. Most disorders can be rarely recognized prenatally.

7.1 Short femur and humerus

On the basis of several studies of cases with shortened long bones (femur and humerus), the incidence rate for the abnormal karyotypes is elevated. According to the literature, a shortened humerus is a more sensitive indicator. Mainly the risk of trisomy 21 increases [114–117].

Studying the long bones, the main ambition of the investigators was to determine the proper method to estimate the measure of the retardation in growth, which increases the risk of chromosome abnormalities. The two main methods are fundamentally different. Some investigators calculate with the observed/expected ratio (O/E ratio) and determine the proper cutoff value by expressing the quotient in percentile (≤0.91) [8, 115]. Other scientists calculate on the basis of the quotient of biparietal diameter (BPD) and femur length (FL) (BPD/FL) and consider abnormal the measure of >1.5 SD [114]. Calculating with both methods, most investigators found significant differences between the fetal groups of normal chromosomes and those with chromosome abnormalities. According to some authors, the difference was not significant [118, 119].

Nyberg et al. [115] examined separately the parameters (O/E ratio) in the case of the humerus and femur and suggested the following cutoff values: humerus ≤0.89 and femur ≤0.91. If both the femur and the humerus are shortened according to the given cutoff values, the risk of trisomy 21 increased 11-fold [115].

Recent studies include both methods. In their report Snijders et al. draw the attention to the fact that although they found significant differences using both methods (O/E ratio, BPD/FL) between fetal groups of normal karyotype and trisomy 21, the screenings before week 18 of gestation are less suitable to predict trisomy 21 [116]. Vergani et al. [117] did not find a significant difference between measuring the O/E ratio and using the BPD/FL method; the difference reached the significance limit ($p = 0.04$). According to their report, the measurement of femur length is connected with the population, and each center should determine the cutoff values dependent on the population on their own [117].

According to a study, chromosome abnormalities occurred in 16% in cases of shortened tubular (long) bones, including 8% of trisomy 18 and 4-4% of monosomy X and trisomy 21 [30].

A Danish publication processed the data of 2718 fetuses detected with shortened femur between the gestational weeks of 17–22, of which 2.5% had chromosome abnormalities. In 11 cases, trisomy 21, in 3 cases trisomy 13, and in 8 cases trisomy 18 were found. Chromosome abnormalities were associated with a higher proportion of these anatomical disorders in the second trimester than the first trimester [120].

7.2 Other abnormalities of the extremities

Other malformations of the extremities increase the risk of trisomy 21 (clinodactyly, widened pelvic angle, sandal gap), trisomy 13 (postaxial polydactyly, clubbed or rocker-bottom feet), and trisomy 18 (clenched hands, overlapping digits, radial aplasia, limb shortening, clubbed feet) [48].

8. Conclusions

Ultrasound examinations play an important role during pregnancy, by drawing the attention to the suspect of a possible abnormality. The prenatal screening of minor ultrasound signs and major ultrasound anomalies and diagnostics is a very important part of the health service. The intrauterine screening and diagnostic methods, the ultrasound screening during the pregnancy, and the cytogenetic and molecular genetic examinations in the genetic centers made the early, intrauterine diagnosis of the chromosomal abnormalities possible.

Conflict of interest

The authors declare no conflict of interest.

Author details

Artúr Beke* and Aténé Simonyi
Department of Obstetrics and Gynaecology, Semmelweis University, Budapest, Hungary

*Address all correspondence to: beke.artur@med.semmelweis-univ.hu

References

[1] Beke A. Ultrasound markers which indicate chromosome analysis. Ultrasound in Obstetrics & Gynecology. 2003;**3**:259-272

[2] Borrell A, Costa D, Martinez JM, Delgado RD, Casals E, Ojuel J, et al. Early midtrimester fetal nuchal thickness: Effectiveness as a marker of down syndrome. American Journal of Obstetrics and Gynecology. 1996;**175**:45-49

[3] Gray DL, Crane JP. Optimal nuchal skin-fold thresholds based on gestational age for prenatal detection of Down syndrome. American Journal of Obstetrics and Gynecology. 1994;**171**:1282-1286

[4] Benacerraf BR, Frigoletto FDJr, Laboda LA. Sonographic diagnosis of down syndrome in the second trimester. American Journal of Obstetrics and Gynecology. 1985;**153**:49-52

[5] Crane JP, Gray DL. Sonographically measured nuchal skinfold thickness as a screening tool for Down syndrome: Results of a prospective clinical trial. Obstetrics and Gynecology. 1991;**77**:533-536

[6] DeVore GR, Alfi O. The association between an abnormal nuchal skin fold, trisomy 21, and ultrasound abnormalities identified during the second trimester of pregnancy. Ultrasound in Obstetrics & Gynecology. 1993;**3**:387-394

[7] Grandjean H, SarramonMF.Sonographicmeasurement of nuchal skinfold thickness for detection of Down syndrome in the second-trimester fetus: A multicenter prospective study. The AFDPHE study group. Association Francaise pour le Depistage et la prevention des Handicaps de l'Enfant. Obstet. Gynécologie. 1995;**85**:103-106

[8] Gonen R, Dar H, Degani S. The karyotype of fetuses with anomalies detected by second trimester ultrasonography. European Journal of Obstetrics, Gynecology, and Reproductive Biology. 1995;**58**:153-155

[9] Zimmer EZ, Drugan A, Ofir C, Blazer S, Bronshtein M. Ultrasound imaging of fetal neck anomalies: Implications for the risk of aneuploidy and structural anomalies. Prenatal Diagnosis. 1997;**17**:1055-1058

[10] Beke A, Joo JG, Csaba A, Lazar L, Ban Z, Papp C, et al. Incidence of chromosomal abnormalities in presence of fetal subcutaneous oedema, nuchal oedema, cystic hygroma and non-immune hydrops. Fetal Diagnosis and Therapy. 2009;**25**:83-92

[11] Azar GB, Snijders RJ, Gosden C, Nicolaides KH. Fetal nuchal cystic hygromata: Associated malformations and chromosomal defects. Fetal Diagnosis and Therapy. 1991;**6**:46-57

[12] Bronshtein M, Bar-Hava I, Blumenfeld I, Bejar J, Toder V, Blumenfeld Z. The difference between septated and nonseptated nuchal cystic hygroma in the early second trimester. Obstetrics and Gynecology. 1993;**81**:683-687

[13] Nadel A, Bromley B, Benacerraf BR. Nuchal thickening or cystic hygromas in first- and early second-trimester fetuses: Prognosis and outcome. Obstetrics and Gynecology. 1993;**82**:43-48

[14] Sohn C, Gast AS. Hygroma colli (cervical neck edema) as an ultrasonographic parameter of fetal chromosome anomalies. Zentralblatt für Gynäkologie. 1997;**119**:232-236

[15] Taipale P, Hiilesmaa V, Salonen R, Ylostalo P. Increased nuchal

translucency as a marker for fetal chromosomal defects. The New England Journal of Medicine. 1997;**337**:1654-1658

[16] Rosati P, Guariglia L. Prognostic value of ultrasound findings of fetal cystic hygroma detected in early pregnancy by transvaginal sonography. Ultrasound in Obstetrics & Gynecology. 2000;**16**:245-250

[17] Tanriverdi HA, Hendrik HJ, Ertan AK, Axt R, Schmidt W. Hygroma colli cysticum: Prenatal diagnosis and prognosis. American Journal of Perinatology. 2001;**18**:415-420

[18] Donnenfeld AE, Lockwood D, Lamb AN. Prenatal diagnosis from cystic hygroma fluid: The value of fluorescence in situ hybridization. American Journal of Obstetrics and Gynecology. 2001;**185**:1004-1008

[19] Gezer C, Ekin A, Gezer NS, Ertas IE, Avci ME, Uyar I, et al. Prenatal karyotype results of fetuses with nuchal edema, cystic hygroma, and non-immune hydrops. Clinical and Experimental Obstetrics & Gynecology. 2015;**42**:586-589

[20] Nicolaides KH, Rodeck CH, Gosden CM. Rapid karyotyping in non-lethal fetal malformations. Lancet. 1986;**1**:283-287

[21] Gembruch U, Hansmann M, Bald R, Zerres K, Schwanitz G, Fodisch HJ. Prenatal diagnosis and management in fetuses with cystic hygromata colli. European Journal of Obstetrics, Gynecology, and Reproductive Biology. 1988;**29**:241-255

[22] Boyd PA, Keeling JW. Fetal hydrops. Journal of Medical Genetics. 1992;**29**:91-97

[23] Anandakumar C, Biswas A, Wong YC, Chia D, Annapoorna V, Arulkumaran S, et al. Management of non-immune hydrops: 8 years' experience. Ultrasound in Obstetrics & Gynecology. 1996;**8**:196-200

[24] Schwanitz G, Zerres K, Gembruch U, Bald R, Hansmann M. Rate of chromosomal aberrations in prenatally detected hydrops fetalis and hygroma colli. Human Genetics. 1989;**84**:81-82

[25] Has R. Non-immune hydrops fetalis in the first trimester: A review of 30 cases. Clinical and Experimental Obstetrics & Gynecology. 2001;**28**:187-190

[26] Patel MD, Goldstein RB, Tung S, Filly RA. Fetal cerebral ventricular atrium: Difference in size according to sex. Radiology. 1995;**194**:713-715

[27] Bromley B, Frigoletto FDJr, Benacerraf BR. Mild fetal lateral cerebral ventriculomegaly: Clinical course and outcome. American Journal of Obstetrics and Gynecology. 1991;**164**:863-867

[28] Mahony BS, Nyberg DA, Hirsch JH, Petty CN, Hendricks SK, Mack LA. Mild idiopathic lateral cerebral ventricular dilatation in utero: Sonographic evaluation. Radiology. 1988;**169**:715-721

[29] Terry M, Calhoun BC, Walker W, Apodaca C, Martin L, Pierce B, et al. Aneuploidy and isolated mild ventriculomegaly. Attributable risk for isolated fetal marker. Fetal Diagnosis and Therapy. 2000;**15**:331-334

[30] Beke A, Papp C, Toth-Pal E, Mezei G, Oroszné NJ, Joo JG, et al. Trisomies and other chromosome abnormalities detected following positive sonographic findings. The Journal of Reproductive Medicine. 2005;**50**:675-691

[31] Ogle RF. Second trimester markers of aneuploidy. Baillière's Best Practice & Research. Clinical Obstetrics & Gynaecology. 2000;**14**:595-610

[32] Snijders RJ, Shawa L, Nicolaides KH. Fetal choroid plexus cysts and trisomy 18: Assessment of risk based on ultrasound findings and maternal age. Prenatal Diagnosis. 1994;**14**:1119-1127

[33] Walkinshaw S, Pilling D, Spriggs A. Isolated choroid plexus cysts—The need for routine offer of karyotyping. Prenatal Diagnosis. 1994;**14**:663-667

[34] Gray DL, Winborn RC, Suessen TL, Crane JP. Is genetic amniocentesis warranted when isolated choroid plexus cysts are found? Prenatal Diagnosis. 1996;**16**:983-990

[35] Turner SR, Samei E, Hertzberg BS, DeLong DM, Vargas-Voracek R, Singer A, et al. Sonography of fetal choroid plexus cysts: Detection depends on cyst size and gestational age. Journal of Ultrasound in Medicine. 2003;**22**:1219-1227

[36] Walkinshaw S. Fetal choroid plexus cysts: Are we there yet? Prenatal Diagnosis. 2000;**20**:657-662

[37] Chudleigh P, Pearce M, Campbell S. The prenatal diagnosis of transient cysts of the fetal choroid plexus. Prenatal Diagnosis. 1984;**4**:135-137

[38] Achiron R, Barkai G, Katznelson MB, Mashiach S. Fetal lateral ventricle choroid plexus cysts: The dilemma of amniocentesis. Obstetrics and Gynecology. 1991;**78**:815-818

[39] Platt LD, Carlson DE, Medearis AL, Walla CA. Fetal choroid plexus cysts in the second trimester of pregnancy: A cause for concern. American Journal of Obstetrics and Gynecology. 1991;**164**:1652-1655

[40] Nadel AS, Bromley BS, Frigoletto FD Jr, Estroff JA, Benacerraf BR. Isolated choroid plexus cysts in the second-trimester fetus: Is amniocentesis really indicated? Radiology. 1992;**185**:545-548

[41] Nava S, Godmilow L, Reeser S, LudomirskyA,DonnenfeldAE.Significance of sonographically detected second-trimester choroid plexus cysts: A series of 211 cases and a review of the literature. Ultrasound in Obstetrics & Gynecology. 1994;**4**:448-451

[42] Bakos O, Moen KS, Hansson S. Prenatal karyotyping of choroid plexus cysts. European Journal of Ultrasound. 1998;**8**:79-83

[43] Chitty LS, Chudleigh P, Wright E, Campbell S, Pembrey M. The significance of choroid plexus cysts in an unselected population: Results of a multicenter study. Ultrasound in Obstetrics & Gynecology. 1998;**12**:391-397

[44] Ghidini A, Strobelt N, Locatelli A, Mariani E, Piccoli MG, Vergani P. Isolated fetal choroid plexus cysts: Role of ultrasonography in establishment of the risk of trisomy 18. American Journal of Obstetrics and Gynecology. 2000;**182**:972-977

[45] Coco C, Jeanty P. Karyotyping of fetuses with isolated choroid plexus cysts is not justified in an unselected population. Journal of Ultrasound in Medicine. 2004;**23**:899-906

[46] Sahinoglu Z, Uludogan M, Sayar C, Turkover B, Toksoy G. Second trimester choroid plexus cysts and trisomy 18. International Journal of Gynaecology and Obstetrics. 2004;**85**:24-29

[47] Beke A, Barakonyi E, Belics Z, Joó JG, Csaba A, Papp C, et al. The risk of chromosome abnormalities in presence of bilateral or unilateral choroid plexus cysts (CPC). Fetal Diagnosis and Therapy. 2008;**23**:185-191

[48] Nyberg DA, Souter VL. Sonographic markers of fetal aneuploidy. Clinincs in Perinatology. 2000;**27**:761-789

[49] Hill LM. The sonographic detection of trisomies 13, 18, and 21. Clinical Obstetrics and Gynecology. 1996;**39**:831-850

[50] Benacerraf BR, Frigoletto FDJr, Bieber FR. The fetal face: Ultrasound examination. Radiology. 1984;**153**:495-497

[51] Parant O, Sarramon MF, Delisle MB, Fournie A. Prenatal diagnosis of holoprosencephaly. A series of twelve cases. Journal de Gynécologie, Obstétrique et Biologie de la Reproduction. 1997;**26**:687-696

[52] Tongsong T, Wanapirak C, Sirichotiyakul S, Siriangkul S. Prenatal sonographic diagnosis of holoprosencephaly. Journal of the Medical Association of Thailand. 1998;**81**:208-213

[53] Bullen PJ, Rankin JM, Robson SC. Investigation of the epidemiology and prenatal diagnosis of holoprosencephaly in the north of England. American Journal of Obstetrics and Gynecology. 2001;**184**:1256-1262

[54] Moog U, De Die-SmuldersCE,Schrander-StumpelCT, Engelen JJ, Hamers AJ, Frints S, et al. Holoprosencephaly: The Maastricht experience. Genetic Counseling. 2001;**12**:287-298

[55] Perrotin F, de Poncheville LM, Marret H, Paillet C, Lansac J, Body G. Chromosomal defects and associated malformations in fetal cleft lip with or without cleft palate. European Journal of Obstetrics, Gynecology, and Reproductive Biology. 2001;**99**:19-24

[56] Aletebi FA, Fung KFK. Neurodevelopmental outcome after antenatal diagnosis of posterior fossa abnormalities. Journal of Ultrasound in Medicine. 1999;**18**:683-689

[57] Nazer Herrera J, Cifuentes Ovalle L, Cortez López A. Frequency of holoprosencephaly in Chile. Revista Médica de Chile. 2015;**143**:874-879

[58] Hayashi Y, Suzumori N, Sugiura T, Sugiura-Ogasawara M. Prenatal findings of holoprosencephaly. Congenital Anomalies. 2015;**55**:161-163

[59] Levy DW, Mintz MC. The left ventricular echogenic focus: A normal finding. American Journal of Roentgenology. 1988;**150**:85-86

[60] Shipp TD, Bromley B, Lieberman E, Benacerraf BR. The frequency of the detection of fetal echogenic intracardiac foci with respect to maternal race. Ultrasound in Obstetrics & Gynecology. 2000;**15**:460-462

[61] Bromley B, Lieberman E, Laboda L, Benacerraf BR. Echogenic intracardiac focus: A sonographic sign for fetal Down syndrome. Obstetrics and Gynecology. 1995;**86**:998-1001

[62] Bromley B, Lieberman E, Shipp TD, Richardson M, Benacerraf BR. Significance of an echogenic intracardiac focus in fetuses at high and low risk for aneuploidy. Journal of Ultrasound in Medicine. 1998;**17**:127-131

[63] Huggon IC, Cook AC, Simpson JM, Smeeton NC, Sharland GK. Isolated echogenic foci in the fetal heart as marker of chromosomal abnormality. Ultrasound in Obstetrics & Gynecology. 2001;**17**:11-16

[64] Sepulveda W, Cullen S, Nicolaidis P, Hollingsworth J, Fisk NM. Echogenic foci in the fetal heart: A marker of chromosomal abnormality. British Journal of Obstetrics and Gynaecology. 1995;**102**:490-492

[65] Winter TC, Anderson AM, Cheng EY, Komarniski CA, Souter VL, Uhrich SB, et al. Echogenic intracardiac focus in 2nd-trimester fetuses with trisomy 21: Usefulness as a US marker. Radiology. 2000;**216**:450-456

[66] Lehman CD, Nyberg DA, Winter TC 3rd, Kapur RP, Resta RG, Luthy DA. Trisomy 13 syndrome: Prenatal US findings in a review of 33 cases. Radiology. 1995;**194**:217-222

[67] Hajdu J, Marton T, Cs P, Cesko I, Oroszne NJ, Papp Z. Prenatal diagnosis of atrioventricular septal defect and its prognostic significance. Orvosi Hetilap. 1998;**139**:23-26

[68] Tennstedt C, Chaoui R, Korner H, Dietel M. Spectrum of congenital heart defects and extracardiac malformations associated with chromosomal abnormalities: Results of a seven year necropsy study. Heart. 1999;**82**:34-39

[69] Delisle MF, Sandor GG, Tessier F, Farquharson DF. Outcome of fetuses diagnosed with atrioventricular septal defect. Obstetrics and Gynecology. 1999;**94**:763-767

[70] Paladini D, Russo M, Teodoro A, Pacileo G, Capozzi G, Martinelli P, et al. Prenatal diagnosis of congenital heart disease in the Naples area during the years 1994-1999—The experience of a joint fetal-pediatric cardiology unit. Prenatal Diagnosis. 2002;**22**:545-552

[71] Hajdu J, Beke A, Pete B, Oroszne NJ, Papp Z. Prenatal diagnosis of the atrioventricular septal defect and it's effect on the outcome of the pregnancies. Orvosi Hetilap. 2005;**146**(34):1775-1780

[72] Bendriss L, Sedrati M, Haddour L, Arharbi M. Ventricular septal defects: Anatomic, clinical, therapeutic and prognostic aspects. 44 cases. Presse Médicale. 2006;**35**(4 Pt 1):593-597

[73] Zhong P, Gu Y, Wang A, Sun X, Wang Y, Zhang X, et al. Complete atrioventricular septal defect: A clinicopathologic study of 35 cases. Zhonghua Bing Li Xue Za Zhi. 2016;**45**:107-110

[74] Shuhaiber JH, Robinson B, Gauvreau K, Breitbart R, Mayer JE, Del Nido PJ, et al. Outcome after repair of atrioventricular septal defect with tetralogy of Fallot. The Journal of Thoracic and Cardiovascular Surgery. 2012;**143**:338-343

[75] Paladini D, Tartaglione A, Agangi A, Teodoro A, Forleo F, Borghese A, et al. The association between congenital heart disease and down syndrome in prenatal life. Ultrasound in Obstetrics & Gynecology. 2000;**15**:104-108

[76] Estoff JA, Parad RB, Frigoletto FD Jr, Benacerraf R. The natural history of isolated fetal hydrothorax. Ultrasound in Obstetrics & Gynecology. 1992;**2**:162-165

[77] Bromley B, Doubilet P, Frigoletto FD Jr, Krauss C, Estroff JA, Benacerraf BR. Is fetal hyperechoic bowel on second-trimester sonogram an indication for amniocentesis? Obstetrics and Gynecology. 1994;**83**:647-651

[78] Nyberg DA, Dubinsky T, Resta RG, Mahony BS, Hickok DE, Luthy DA. Echogenic fetal bowel during the second trimester: Clinical importance. Radiology. 1993;**188**:527-531

[79] Scioscia AL, Pretorius DH, Budorick NE, Cahill TC, Axelrod FT, Leopold GR. Second-trimester echogenic bowel and chromosomal abnormalities. American Journal of Obstetrics and Gynecology. 1992;**167**:889-894

[80] Strocker AM, Snijders RJ, Carlson DE, Greene N, Gregory KD, Walla CA, et al. Fetal echogenic bowel:

Parameters to be considered in differential diagnosis. Ultrasound in Obstetrics & Gynecology. 2000;**16**:519-523

[81] Sipes SL, Weiner CP, Wenstrom KD, Williamson RA, Grant SS, Mueller GM. Fetal echogenic bowel on ultrasound: Is there clinical significance? Fetal Diagnosis and Therapy. 1994;**9**:38-43

[82] Blancato JK, Hunt M, George J, Katz J, Meck JM. Prenatal diagnosis of tetrasomy 12p by in situ hybridization: Varying levels of mosaicism in different fetal tissues. Prenatal Diagnosis. 1992;**12**:979-983

[83] Donnenfeld AE, Campbell TJ, Byers J, Librizzi RJ, Weiner S. Tissue-specific mosaicism among fetuses with prenatally diagnosed diaphragmatic hernia. American Journal of Obstetrics and Gynecology. 1993;**169**:1017-1021

[84] Huddy CL, Boyd PA, Wilkinson AR, Chamberlain P. Congenital diaphragmatic hernia: Prenatal diagnosis, outcome and continuing morbidity in survivors. British Journal of Obstetrics and Gynaecology. 1999;**106**:1192-1196

[85] Mann L, Ferguson-Smith MA, Desai M, Gibson AA, Raine PA. Prenatal assessment of anterior abdominal wall defects and their prognosis. Prenatal Diagnosis. 1984;**4**:427-435

[86] Rabe D, Hendrik HJ, Leucht W, Roth H, Walter C, Schmidt W. Ventral abdominal wall defects—Antenatal diagnosis, course of pregnancy and post partum therapy. Geburtshilfe und Frauenheilkunde. 1985;**45**:176-182

[87] Gilbert WM, Nicolaides KH. Fetal omphalocele: Associated malformations and chromosomal defects. Obstetrics and Gynecology. 1987;**70**:633-635

[88] Nyberg DA, Fitzsimmons J, Mack LA, Hughes M, Pretorius DH, Hickok D, et al. Chromosomal abnormalities in fetuses with omphalocele. Significance of omphalocele contents. Journal of Ultrasound in Medicine. 1989;**8**:299-308

[89] Holzgreve W, Miny P, Gerlach B, Westendorp A, Ahlert D, Horst J. Benefits of placental biopsies for rapid karyotyping in the second and third trimesters (late chorionic villus sampling) in high-risk pregnancies. American Journal of Obstetrics and Gynecology. 1990;**162**:1188-1192

[90] Rizzo N, Pittalis MC, Pilu G, Orsini LF, Perolo A, Bovicelli L. Prenatal karyotyping in malformed foetuses. Prenatal Diagnosis. 1990;**10**:17-23

[91] Fogel M, Copel JA, Cullen MT, Hobbins JC, Kleinman CS. Congenital heart disease and fetal thoracoabdominal anomalies: Associations in utero and the importance of cytogenetic analysis. American Journal of Perinatology. 1991;**8**:411-416

[92] Nicolaides KH, Snijders RJ, Cheng HH, Gosden C. Fetal gastro-intestinal and abdominal wall defects: Associated malformations and chromosomal abnormalities. Fetal Diagnosis and Therapy. 1992;**7**:102-115

[93] Snijders RJ, Brizot ML, Faria M, Nicolaides KH. Fetal exomphalos at 11 to 14 weeks of gestation. Journal of Ultrasound in Medicine. 1995;**14**:569-574

[94] Dillon E, Renwick M. The antenatal diagnosis and management of abdominal wall defects: The northern region experience. Clinical Radiology. 1995;**50**:855-859

[95] Axt R, Quijano F, Boos R, Hendrik HJ, Jessberger HJ, Schwaiger C, et al. Omphalocele and gastroschisis: Prenatal diagnosis and peripartal management. A case analysis of the years 1989-1997 at the Department of

Obstetrics and Gynecology, University of Homburg/Saar. European Journal of Obstetrics, Gynecology, and Reproductive Biology. 1999;**87**:47-54

[96] Rankin J, Dillon E, Wright C. Congenital anterior abdominal wall defects in the north of England, 1986-1996: Occurrence and outcome. Prenatal Diagnosis. 1999;**19**:662-668

[97] Stoll C, Alembik Y, Dott B, Roth MP. Risk factors in congenital abdominal wall defects (omphalocele and gastroschisis): A study in a series of 265,858 consecutive births. Annales de Génétique. 2001;**44**:201-208

[98] Barisic I, Clementi M, Hausler M, Gjergja R, Kern J, Stoll C, et al., Euroscan Study Group. Evaluation of prenatal ultrasound diagnosis of fetal abdominal wall defects by 19 European registries. Ultrasound in Obstetrics & Gynecology. 2001;**18**:309-316

[99] Salihu HM, Boos R, Schmidt W. Omphalocele and gastrochisis. Journal of Obstetrics and Gynaecology. 2002;**22**:489-492

[100] Ozawa K, Ishikawa H, Maruyama Y, Nagata T, Nagase H, Itani Y, et al. Congenital omphalocele and polyhydramnios: A study of 52 cases. Fetal Diagnosis and Therapy. 2011;**30**:184-188

[101] Stoll C, Alembik Y, Dott B, Roth MP. Omphalocele and gastroschisis and associated malformations. American Journal of Medical Genetics. Part A. 2008;**146A**:1280-1285

[102] Bailey PV, Tracy TFJr, Connors RH, Mooney DP, Lewis JE, Weber TR. Congenital duodenal obstruction: A 32-year review. Journal of Pediatric Surgery. 1993;**28**:92-95

[103] Heydanus R, Spaargaren MC, Wladimiroff JW. Prenatal ultrasonic diagnosis of obstructive bowel disease: A retrospective analysis. Prenatal Diagnosis. 1994;**14**:1035-1041

[104] Lawrence MJ, Ford WD, Furness ME, Hayward T, Wilson T. Congenital duodenal obstruction: Early antenatal ultrasound diagnosis. Pediatric Surgery International. 2000;**16**:342-345

[105] Nyberg DA, Resta RG, Luthy DA, Hickok DE, Mahony BS, Hirsch JH. Prenatal sonographic findings of down syndrome, review of 94 cases. Obstetrics and Gynecology. 1990;**76**:370-377

[106] Slotnick RN, Abuhamad AZ. Prognostic implications of fetal echogenic bowel. Lancet. 1996;**347**:85-87

[107] Benacerraf BR, Mandell J, Estroff JA, Harlow BL, Frigoletto FD. Fetal pyelectasis: A possible association with Down syndrome. Obstetrics and Gynecology. 1990;**76**:58-60

[108] Chudleigh PM, Chitty L, Pembrey M, Campbell S. The association of aneuploidy and mild fetal pyelectasis in an unselected population: The results of a multicenter study. Ultrasound in Obstetrics & Gynecology. 2001;**17**:197-202

[109] Corteville JE, Dicke JM, Crane JP. Fetal pyelectasis and down syndrome: Is genetic amniocentesis warranted? Obstetrics and Gynecology. 1992;**79**:770-772

[110] Wilson RD, Lynch S, Lessoway VA. Fetal pyelectasis: Comparison of postnatal renal pathology with unilateral and bilateral pyelectasis. Prenatal Diagnosis. 1997;**17**:451-455

[111] Wickstrom E, Maizels M, Sabbagha RE, Tamura RK, Cohen LC, Pergament E. Isolated fetal pyelectasis:

Assessment of risk for postnatal uropathy and down syndrome. Ultrasound in Obstetrics & Gynecology. 1996;**8**:236-240

[112] Bronstein E, Barnhard Y, Donnenfeld A, Ferber A, Divon MY. Fetal pyelectasis: Does fetal gender modify the risk of major trisomies? Obstetrics and Gynecology. 2006;**107**:877-879

[113] Coco C, Jeanty P. Isolated fetal pyelectasis and chromosomal abnormalities. American Journal of Obstetrics and Gynecology. 2005;**93**:732-738

[114] Johnson MP, Michaelson JE, Barr M Jr, Treadwell MC, Hume RF Jr, Dombrowski MP, et al. Combining humerus and femur length for improved ultrasonographic identification of pregnancies at increased risk for trisomy 21. American Journal of Obstetrics and Gynecology. 1995;**172**:1229-1235

[115] Nyberg DA, Resta RG, Luthy DA, Hickok DE, Williams MA. Humerus and femur length shortening in the detection of Down's syndrome. American Journal of Obstetrics and Gynecology. 1993;**168**:534-538

[116] Snijders RJ, Platt LD, Greene N, Carlson D, Krakow D, Gregory K, et al. Femur length and trisomy 21: Impact of gestational age on screening efficiency. Ultrasound in Obstetrics & Gynecology. 2000;**16**:142-145

[117] Vergani P, Locatelli A, Piccoli MG, Mariani E, Strobelt N, Pezzullo JC, et al. Critical reappraisal of the utility of sonographic fetal femur length in the prediction of trisomy 21. Prenatal Diagnosis. 2000;**20**:210-214

[118] Perrella R, Duerinckx AJ, Grant EG, Tessler F, Tabsh K, Crandall BF. Second-trimester sonographic diagnosis of down syndrome: Role of femur-length shortening and nuchal-fold thickening. AJR. American Journal of Roentgenology. 1988;**151**:981-985

[119] LaFollette L, Filly R, Anderson R, Golbus MS. Fetal femur length to detect trisomy 21. A reappraisal. Journal of Ultrasound in Medicine. 1989;**8**:657-660

[120] Mathiesen JM, Aksglaede L, Skibsted L, Petersen OB, Tabor A, Danish Fetal Medicine Study Group. Outcome of fetuses with short femur length detected at second-trimester anomaly scan: A national survey. Ultrasound in Obstetrics & Gynecology. 2014;**44**:160-165

Chapter 3

Impact of Biological Factors Related to Maternal Aging: Risk of Childbirth with Down Syndrome

Subrata Kumar Dey, Pranami Bhaumik and Mandar Bhattacharya

Abstract

Maternal aging and different biological factors play an important role in the birth of Down syndrome baby. Hormones play a crucial role for the maintenance of female sex cycle and oocyte maturation. Disparity in the level of these hormones during menstrual cycle has profound effect on female reproductive system. Hormonal imbalance also affects meiotic process and integrity of spindle structure and leads to nondisjunction of chromosome. Follicle-stimulating hormone (FSH), anti-Müllerian hormone (AMH) and luteinizing hormone (LH) play a crucial role in ovarian aging and nondisjunction of chromosomes. FSH stands as a hormonal indicator for ovarian aging, and its high level is responsible for aneuploid birth. Advanced chronological age of mother, ovarian aging, environmental factors and accelerated telomere shortening at older reproductive age are found to be risk factors for the birth of trisomy 21 Down syndrome.

Keywords: hormones, ovarian aging, nondisjunction, Down syndrome, trisomy 21, oocyte, telomere

1. Introduction

Down syndrome (DS), the most frequent live born aneuploidy in human, is predominantly caused by trisomy of chromosome 21 (Ch21), and its etiologic factors are under continuous scrutiny since its discovery by Lejeune et al. [1]. Several groups of workers have tried to explore the factors associated with nondisjunction (NDJ) of Ch21 and have identified that advanced maternal age [2, 3] and altered pattern of recombination are two strong correlates that affect proper segregation of chromosomes at oogenesis, particularly at first meiotic division (MI) [2, 4]. In elucidating the important causes of these sex bias risk factors, two hypotheses have been suggested. According to one school of thought [4], the extended phase of MI arrest in women that lasts for several years makes the oocyte more vulnerable to NDJ than spermatozoa. On the other hand, other investigators emphasized the meiotic drive of chromosomes and subsequent natural selection in asymmetric meiosis in females as the probable reasons of sex biasness of NDJ [5]. The association of advanced maternal age with DS birth is still an enigma. Although advanced maternal age is not the cause of NDJ, it is an obvious risk of DS birth. The overall maternal risk for DS birth is suggested to be multifactorial and includes both genetic and environmental factors [2, 4, 6, 7] that impart adverse effects in either an age-dependent manner or a stochastic age-unrelated fashion [8]. In addition to genetic correlates, the genotoxic effects of smoking, chewing tobacco and oral contraceptive pills on reproductive health and fertility have also been investigated [9]. All these risk factors exacerbate age-related maternal risk for the birth of DS babies [10–12]. Telomere length is a powerful biomarker for aging. Telomere erosion at advanced reproductive age might affect the chromosomal segregation during oogenesis, and there is a strong relation between maternal aging and telomere length attrition [7, 13].

1.1 Hormonal imbalance with aging

A complex orchestrated hormonal cascade plays a very crucial role for the maintenance of female sex cycle and oocyte maturation. The brain hypothalamus releases luteinizing hormone-releasing hormone (LHRH) that triggers the anterior pituitary gland to release follicle-stimulating hormone (FSH) and luteinizing hormone (LH). FSH and LH in turn stimulate ovary to produce estrogen (mainly estradiol) and progesterone using an complicated feedback loop. Disparities in the level of these hormones during menstrual cycle have a profound effect on female reproductive system. They are responsible for the recommencement of meiosis I in the oocyte [14], change in the follicular micro-environment around oocytes and prepare the endometrial layer of uterus for implantation of fertilized ovum [15, 16]. Maturity of oocyte, rate of meiosis and integrity of spindle are disturbed by imbalanced level of hormones and eventually lead to nondisjunction [17–19]. However, there are two major hormones FSH and anti-Müllerian hormone serve as powerful biomarkers of ovarian aging.

1.2 Follicle-stimulating hormone (FSH), aging and aneuploid birth

FSH plays a crucial role in nondisjunction. It has been documented that FSH level rises with ovarian aging [20, 21]. Moreover, women giving birth to Down syndrome (DS) child are reported to have elevated FSH level [22, 23], indicating the effect of aging on the oocyte pool. Demonstrated that higher concentration of FSH evokes chromosomal aneuploidy in murine model. They showed that the elevated FSH hampers chromosomal alignment in prometaphase and metaphase stages of meiosis I and gives rise to aneuploid oocyte. Granulosa cells of maturing follicles exclusively possess FSH receptors that are linked directly to oocyte with gap junctions [24, 25]. Thus, the effect of FSH on cumulus cells directly conducted to oocytes via secondary messenger cAMP and downstream kinase cascade [26, 27]. The spindle formation, its assembly and number of centromere in oocyte are perturbed by adverse effect of FSH both *in vivo* and *in vitro* [28]. It is also apparent that age-related reproductive failure is accelerated in transgenic FSH mice [29]. Researchers hypothesized that FSH alters the intra follicular environment that either facilitates the recruitment of an error-prone oocyte or affects cohesins and in turn reduce the pairing ability of chromosomes. Thus, chronic exposure to high FSH promotes rapid depletion of oocyte pool and accounts for trisomic pregnancies [30]. These evidences suggest that FSH stands as a hormonal indicator of ovarian aging, and its high level is responsible for aneuploid birth.

1.3 Anti-Müllerian hormone (AMH), ovarian reserve and aneuploid birth

Anti-Müllerian hormone (AMH) or Müllerian inhibiting substance (MIS) is a homodimeric glycoprotein and belongs to transforming growth factor-β (TGF-β) superfamily. Synthesis of AMH occurs in ovarian granulosa cells. Several studies exhibit its prime role as a useful biomarker for ovarian reserve [31–34]. Gradual aging affirms a decline in the level of serum AMH. This hormone is proved to be a superior predictor of ovarian reserve than chronological age [35, 36]. The quality of an embryo depends upon both the quantity and quality of ovarian reserve which diminished with age. AMH, however, is essential for the maintenance of both the number and functional quality of oocyte pool. Moreover, AMH is a stable marker and not influenced by pregnancy, oral contraceptives and antagonist of gonadotropin-releasing hormone [37–41]. The undetectable level of AMH after 3–5 days of bilateral ovariectomy suggests that the origin of the circulating AMH is chiefly ovarian [39, 40]. AMH is an exclusive endocrine parameter to presume the ovarian function as it is evident from several studies that AMH level remains mostly unchanged throughout menstrual cycle unlike other gonadotropins and steroids [38, 42–44]. The association between serum AMH and fetal aneuploidy is a topic of debate. Seifer and Maclaughlin found lack of association of maternal AMH and Down syndrome conceptions [34]. This finding was again supported by Plante et al. who suggested that AMH decreases with age, and the dose level did not vary in cases of aneuploid and euploid pregnancies [45]; whereas Shim et al. demonstrated a significant association of circulating AMH with fetal aneuploidy in early pregnancies [46].

2. Alteration of sister chromatid cohesion: aging effect

A growing body of evidence suggests that aneuploid fetus formation speeds up as maternal age crosses 35 years. Moreover, a 10-fold increase in aneuploid conception is apparent after 38 years and involves aneuploidy of multiple chromosomes [47–49]. In older women, the probability of erroneous separation of sister centromere increases in anaphase-II [47, 48, 50]. Extensive loss of centromeric cohesion and subsequent instability of spindle are reported in oocytes arrested in MII from aged women [51–53]. Cohesin protein between two sister chromatids depletes with aging and gives rise to nondisjunction error [54]. Studies reveal that in MII oocytes of older mice [55, 56] and women [57], sister chromatids having incompletely separated distantly placed centromeres face problem in biorientation and result in spindle instability.

3. Telomere theory of ovarian aging

The telomeres are the nucleotide repeat sequence TTAGGG insulating the terminal ends of eukaryotic chromosomes, protecting them from getting fused with adjacent chromosomes [58]. In each cell division, telomere corrodes and restored by a unique reverse transcriptase called telomerase [59]. Gradual depletion of telomere length with age marked it as an impressive biomarker of aging [60]. Ovarian aging confirms a positive correlation between shorter telomere length and decreased reproductive lifespan [61]. The role of telomere biology in reproduction is supported by numerous opinions. Telomere theory of reproductive senescence states that prolonged exposure to reactive oxygen species (ROS) hastens the erosion of telomere in older women [62]. Telomerase is imperative for oocyte development and parthenogenesis. Telomerase is found in early antral follicle, preovulatory follicle and ovulated oocyte, but its expression diminishes at the time of oocyte maturation [63, 64]. After fertilization, telomerase activity ensures remodeling of telomere length (TL) essential for faithful embryonic development.

A conversed correlation exists amid the activity of telomerase and ovarian aging [65]. In occult ovarian insufficiency, telomerase inactivation and erosion of telomere are evident [66]. Researchers showed that telomere-deficient mice are infertile [67, 68]. Ovarian and uterine malformation and inadequacy of steroid hormone are apparent in mice lacking telomerase [68]. Oocytes having shorter telomere undergo aberrant fertilization and bizarre pattern of embryonic cleavage [69]. Age-related abrasion of telomere may in turn responsible for age-related aneuploidy. Mania et al. [70] exhibited that the aneuploid cells derived from disorganized cleavage-stage embryos have shorter telomeres than euploid cells in mother with older reproductive age or with recurrent history of miscarriage. Telomere shortening is also associated with aneuploidy in malignant cells [71]. Dorland et al. did not find any significant difference in telomere length between mothers of Down syndrome babies and euploid children [72]. However, Ghosh et al. and Bhaumik et al. demonstrated that the older mothers of Down syndrome child have shorter telomere than control [7, 13]. The author suggested that there is a perceptive connection between the constituents of telomere maintenance machinery and chromosome segregation system at molecular level. Moreover, this speculation is supported by several studies stating that disturbed telomere protection is responsible for chromosomal missegregation [73, 74]. Again, in yeast *Saccharomyces cerevisiae*, the improper chromosome separation was noticed due to mutant telomere sequence [75]. Thus, telomere biology has a great impact on the reproductive success particularly in nondisjunction.

3.1 Ovarian aging: genetic background

There is an enigma about the factors influencing the age at menopause in women. Certain lifestyle factors like parity, use of oral contraceptive pills and smoking habits are reported to be pertinent with the age of natural menopause [76]. However, discrepancy in menopausal age cannot be fully interpreted by these factors [77]. Growing body of research indicate that "menopausal age" is a complex genetic trait regulated by genetic factors. This notion is supported by the associations between menopausal age of mother-daughter pairs and sister pairs [78–80]. Premature ovarian failure (POF) is considered as a study model of ovarian aging. Researches revealed that several genetic variations are associated with POF [81, 82]. Variations in genes encoding sex hormones (FSH, FSHR, LH, LHR), enzymes (CYP17, CYP19) and those responsible for follicular recruitment (BMP15, GDF9, and GPR3) regulate the durability of oocyte pool and in turn adjust the span of reproductive life [83]. POF patients are also reported to carry mutations in genes (NANOS, GDF9, NOBOX, LDX8, etc.) expressed in the course of oogenesis [84]. Gene copy number variations (CNVs) are also linked to POF manifestation [85–88]. Gene involved in maturation of primary follicles, apoptosis of follicles, fetal ovarian development or vascularization in ovary are the suitable candidates for studying genetic background of POF [89–92]. Menopausal age is also associated with the presence of mutant allele factor V Leiden or E2 allele of apolipoprotein E [93–95]. Gene-driven compromised microcirculation around oocyte pool is considered as a prime cause of early menopause [96]. Studies pointed out that polymorphisms in genes playing role in steroidogenic pathways like 5-α-reductase type 2 [97] and CYP1B1 [98] also regulate menopausal age. However, polymorphism in folate pathway genes like MTHFR or MTRR is also associated with POF phenotype [99, 100] as well as with trisomy 21 conception [101–104]. Genome-wide association studies identified powerful association between menopausal age and variations in chromosome numbers 20, 19, 5, 6 and 13 [105, 106].

4. Molecular factors associated with maternal age

Advanced chronological age of mother is probably the oldest known factor associated with Down syndrome birth. Risk of having a trisomy 21 baby significantly increases as mother ages. This advanced chronological aging was first postulated in the year of 1933 [107]. Advanced maternal age-specific Down syndrome birth has been studied in almost all the population. One interesting point that came up from these studies is that maternal age varies with the type of nondisjunction. Ages of MII error mother are on the right side to that of MI mothers. Therefore, chronological aging has a direct impact on not only the origin of the disease as well as disease subgroups. Some studies proposed halting of meiosis during oogenesis exert a negative impact on the oocytes. Female oocytes unlike male sperm undergo several checkpoints halting during maturation as meiosis I occur only during puberty and meiosis II after fertilization. This prolonged inertness of oocyte might make it vulnerable to aging-related deterioration. Accumulation of stress factors over time may disrupt the proper chromosomal segregation machinery inducing nondisjunction. Cohesion proteins were expressed during intrauterine condition and must remain active till the completion of meiosis. During this period (~50 years), any disruption in cohesin machinery will result in nondisjunction [108]. Separase cleaves cohesin to release the bound chromatids. Shugoshin-mediated cohesin protection therefore plays a major role in premature separation of sister chromatids (PSSC) [109, 110]. In mice model, age-specific loosening of SMC1beta is observed resulting in abnormal chromosomal segregation [111]. Percentage of premature sister chromatid separation increases in a six-month SMC1b−/− old mother compared to a 1-month-old mother. Age-specific cohesion loosening is also present in *Drosophila* [112]. However, whether age-dependent deterioration or replacement of cohesin is affected by progressive maternal age is still up for debate [113]. Not only cohesin proteins, mitotic proteins associated with spindle assembly are also affected by aging process. Oocytes from older mice have significantly lower expression of MCAK mRNA with altered AURKB [114]. MAD, BUB and TTK are also proposed to decline with progressive aging [115–119]. However, there are alternate studies where it has been proposed that SAC components have similar effect on both old and young oocytes [120]. Therefore, initial cohesion loosening may not recruit MCAK to centromere, properly disrupting normal microtubule depolymerization process [121].

Putting aside chronological aging effect on meiotic machinery, separate model proposes genetic aging as the origin of aneuploidy. Using telomere length as marker, older Down syndrome bearing mother showed rapid telomere attrition than their younger counterpart. Therefore, only older mother experiences this genetic aging. However, we need to keep in mind that peripheral telomere length might not be an actual interpreter of oocytes telomere length. This hypothesis proposes a separate theory about the origin of aneuploidy which was proposed in the year of 1989. Ovarian follicles are formed during intrauterine period in female fetuses. Once puberty is reached, usually one follicle becomes antral follicle and after maturation, ovulates. Total number of follicles and selectable follicles go down as females' age. There may be couple of thousands of follicles present at the age around 40, only two to three selectable follicles present in both the ovaries [122, 123]. Therefore, as women age, the chance of suboptimal follicle ovulation increases [19, 124].

4.1 Recombination pattern and frequency of association with maternal age

Maternal nondisjunction is a multifactorial phenomenon. One major factor that contributes to NDJ is altered recombination pattern during meiosis [125].

Chiasmata is the physical connection where two non-sister chromatids exchange genetic materials in first meiotic division. They stabilize sister chromatids, ensure proper chromosomal spindle attachments and segregation [126]. However, absence of chiasma leads to a situation where chromosomes freely move around, increasing the possibility of aneuploidy. Not only is the absence of chiasma, placement of chiasma is equally important. Achismate condition gives rise to MI meiotic errors. Single telomeric chiasma is an important risk factor for MI type meiotic error as well. Pericentromeric chiasma formation, on the other hand, increases MII meiotic error risk. A broad array of studies conducted with several model organisms such as *Drosophila* [127–129], yeast [130, 131] and *Caenorhabditis elegans* [132] support this fact. In the light of chromosome 21 specific nondisjunction, absence of chiasma formation is a major cause of recombination frequency reduction [133]. Low percentage of detectable crossovers in Ch21 NDJ has been observed across different population [4, 134]. About 57% reductions in linkage map length were reported in Indian population [30.8 cM compared to 72.1 cM CEPH] [6]. Association between advanced chronological age and recombination frequency reduction is well known [135]. 21q-specific recombination analysis showed lower percentage of recombination in older mothers (aged 35 or higher) compared to younger mother [135]. Therefore, absence of recombination could be an age-dependent factor. Studies conducted on Indian population revealed 80% of younger mothers are achismate and had MI NDJ [134]. STR analysis of trisomy 21 families showed high number of single telomeric exchanges in MI NDJ mothers and higher number of single centromeric exchange in MII NDJ mothers. A hypothesis proposed by Ghosh et al. stated that telomeric chiasma as maternal age-independent risk, whereas pericentromeric chiasma is age dependent. How pericentromeric chiasma is affected by maternal age is debatable. Two possible models have been proposed. In the first model, pericentromeric chromosomal exchange may trigger different configurations which increase susceptibility to age-related risk. In the second model, pericentromeric exchange may allow proper segregation in MI but not in MII [8]. As previously mentioned, age-related degradation of cohesion machinery may be a reason behind abnormal chiasma formation. Unlike pericentromeric exchanges, telomeric exchanges give rise to MI type NDJ. The proper reason behind it is not clear. One reason might be the lower amount of cohesion complex in distal region. In Indian cohort, the single chiasma formation was scored at near telomeric 5.1 Mb region [134]. Therefore, single telomeric chiasma can up the risk of NDJ of Ch21 irrespective of maternal age. Lack of biorientation of homologs due to low cohesion protein can give rise to single telomeric chiasma error [127]. Number of studies conducted on different chromosomes showed linear relationship between maternal age and chiasma frequency [136–138]. Multiple chiasmas may increase bivalent stability during MI; therefore, NDJ might not occur.

5. Conclusion

Down syndrome birth is attributable to multiple maternal risk factors that include both genetic and environmental challenges, but there is limited understanding of the complicated interactions among these factors. Along with aging-induced hormonal imbalance, environmental factors such as cigarette smoking, oral contraceptive pills, consumption of alcohol, and use of smokeless chewing tobacco interact with molecular components of the oocyte which ultimately increase the risk of chromosome 21 nondisjunction and subsequently of giving birth to a child with Down syndrome. Age-related abrasion of telomere may in turn be responsible for age-related meiotic abnormalities, subsequent aneuploidy and birth of DS babies in genetically older mother. This "genetic aging" is probably the background cause of all age-related degenerative changes and malfunctions in the ovary.

Author details

Subrata Kumar Dey*, Pranami Bhaumik and Mandar Bhattacharya
Department of Biotechnology, Centre for Genetic Studies, Maulana Abul Kalam Azad University of Technology (Formerly West Bengal University of Technology), Kolkata, West Bengal, India

*Address all correspondence to: subratadey184@gmail.com

References

[1] Lejeune J, Turpin R, Gautier M. Mongolism: A chromosomal disease (trisomy). Bulletin de l Academie Nationale de Medecine. 1959;**143**:256-265

[2] Allen EG, Freeman SB, Druschel C, Hobbs CA, O'Leary LA, Romitti PA, et al. Maternal age and risk for trisomy21 assessed by the origin of chromosome nondisjunction: A report from the Atlanta and National Down Syndrome Projects. Human Genetics. 2009;**125**:41-52

[3] Hassold T, Chiu D. Maternal age specific rates of numerical chromosome abnormalities with special reference to trisomy. Human Genetics. 1985;**70**:11-17

[4] Sherman SL, Allen EG, Bean LH, Freeman SB. Epidemiology of Down syndrome. Mental Retardation and Developmental Disabilities Research Reviews. 2007;**13**:221-227

[5] Zwick ME, Salstrom JL, Langley CH. Genetic variation in rates of nondisjunction: Association of two naturally occurring polymorphisms in the chromokinesin nod with increased rates of nondisjunction in *Drosophila melanogaster*. Genetics. 1999;**152**:1605-1614

[6] Ghosh S, Feingold E, Chakraborty S, Dey SK. Telomere length is associated with types of chromosome 21 NDJ: A new insight into the maternal age effect on Down syndrome birth. Human Genetics. 2010;**127**:403-409

[7] Ghosh S, Bhaumik P, Ghosh P, Dey SK. Chromosome 21 nondisjunction and Down syndrome birth in Indian cohort: Analysis of incidence and etiology from family linkage data. Genetics Research. 2010;**92**:189-197

[8] Oliver TR, Feingold E, Yu K, Cheung V, Tinker S, Yadav-Shah M, et al. New insights into human nondisjunction of chromosome 21 in oocytes. PLOS Genetics. 2008;**4**:e1000033

[9] Ghosh S, Hong C-S, Feingold E, Ghosh P, Ghosh P, Bhaumik P, et al. Epidemiology of Down syndrome: New insight into the multidimensional interactions among genetic and environmental risk factors in the oocyte. American Journal of Epidemiology. 2011;**10**:1-8

[10] Hook EB, Cross PK. Maternal cigarette smoking, Down syndrome in live births, and infant race. American Journal of Human Genetics. 1988;**42**(30):482-489

[11] Kallen K. Downs syndrome and maternal smoking in early pregnancy. Genetic Epidemiology. 1997;**14**(1):77-84

[12] Trofor A, Man MA, Miron R. Smoking during pregnancy—A challenge to practitioners. Pneumologia. 2009;**58**(4):247-249 251

[13] Bhaumik P, Bhattacharya M, Ghosh P, Ghosh S, Kumar Dey S. Telomere length analysis in Down syndrome birth. Mechanisms of Ageing and Development. 2017;**164**:20-26

[14] Crowley PH, Gulati DK, Hayden TL, Lopez P, Dyer R. A chiasma-hormonal hypothesis relating Down's syndrome and maternal age. Nature. 1979;**280**(5721):417-418

[15] Guyton A. Textbook of Medical Physiology. 8th ed. New York: Harcourt Brace Jovanovich; 1991. pp. 826-899

[16] Moore K. The Developing Human. 4th ed. New York: Harcourt Brace Jovanovich; 1988. p. 167

[17] Eichenlaub-Ritter U, Boll I. Nocodazole sensitivity, age-related aneuploidy and alterations in the cell cycle during maturation of mouse oocytes. Cytogenetics and Cell Genetics. 1989;**52**:170-176

[18] Gaulden M. Maternal age effect: The enigma of Down syndrome and other trisomic conditions. Mutation Research. 1992;**296**:69-88

[19] Warburton D. The effect of maternal age on the frequency of trisomy: Change in meiosis or in utero selection? Progress in Clinical and Biological Research. 1989;**311**:165-181

[20] Klein NA, Battaglia DE, Fujimoto VY, Davis GS, Bremner WJ, Soules MR. Reproductive aging: Accelerated ovarian follicular development associated with a monotropic follicle-stimulating hormone rise in normal older women. The Journal of Clinical Endocrinology and Metabolism. 1996;**81**:1038-1045

[21] Santoro N, Brown JR, Adel T, Skurnick JH. Characterization of reproductive hormonal dynamics in the perimenopause. Journal of Clinical Endocrinology and Metabolism. 1996;**81**:1495-1501

[22] Nasseri A, Mukherjee T, Grifo JA, Noyes N, Krey L, Copperman AB. Elevated day 3 serum follicle stimulating hormone and/or estradiol may predict fetalaneuploidy. Fertility and Sterility. 1999;**71**(4):715-718

[23] van Montfrans JM, Dorland M, Oosterhuis GJ, van Vugt JM, Rekers-Mombarg LT, Lambalk CB. Increased concentrations of follicle-stimulating hormone in mothers of children with Down's syndrome. Lancet. 1999;**353**(9167):1853-1854

[24] Albertini DF, Anderson E. The appearance and structure of intercellular connections during the ontogeny of the rabbit ovarian follicle with particular reference to gap junctions. The Journal of Cell Biology. 1974;**63**:234-250

[25] Anderson E, Albertini DF. Gap junctions between the oocyte and companion follicle cells in the mammalian ovary. The Journal of Cell Biology. 1976;**71**:680-686

[26] Gonzalez-Robayna IJ, Falender AE, Ochsner S, Firestone GL, Richards JS. Follicle-stimulating hormone (FSH) stimulates phosphorylation and activation of protein kinase B (PKB/Akt) and serum and glucocorticoid-induced kinase (Sgk): Evidence for a kinase-independent signaling by FSH in granulosa cells. Molecular Endocrinology. 2000;**14**:1283-1300

[27] Richards JS. New signaling pathways for hormones and cyclic adenosine 39,59-monophosphate action in endocrine cells. Molecular Endocrinology. 2001;**15**:209-218

[28] Albertini DF. Cytoplasmic microtubular dynamics and chromatin organization during mammalian oogenesis and oocyte maturation. Mutation Research. 1992;**296**:57-68

[29] McTavish KJ, Jimenez M, Walters KA, Spaliviero J, Groome NP, Themmen AP, et al. Rising follicle-stimulating hormone levels with age accelerate female reproductive failure. Endocrinology. 2007;**148**:4432-4439

[30] Kline JK, Kinney AM, Levin B, Kelly AC, Ferin M, Warburton D. Trisomic pregnancy and elevated FSH: Implications for the oocyte pool hypothesis. Human Reproduction. 2011;**26**(6):1537-1550

[31] Hassold T, Hunt P. To err (meiotically) is human: The genesis of human aneuploidy. Nature Reviews. Genetics. 2001;**2**:280-291

[32] Jayaprakasan K, Campbell B, HopkissonJ,JohnsonI,Raine-FenningN.A prospective, comparative analysis of anti-Müllerian hormone, inhibin-B, and three-dimensional ultrasound determinants of ovarian reserve in the prediction of poor response to controlled ovarian stimulation. Fertility and Sterility. 2010;**93**:855-864

[33] Josso N, Picard JY, Rey R, di Clemente N. Testicular anti-Mullerian hormone: History, genetics, regulation and clinical applications. Pediatric Endocrinology Reviews. 2006;**3**:347-358

[34] Seifer DB, Maclaughlin DT. Mullerian inhibiting substance is an ovarian growth factor of emerging clinical significance. Fertility and Sterility. 2007;**88**:539-546

[35] de Vet A, Laven JS, de Jong FH, Themmen AP, Fauser BC. Antimullerian hormone serum levels: A putative marker for ovarian aging. Fertility and Sterility. 2002;**77**:357-362

[36] van Rooij IA, Broekmans FJ, Scheffer GJ, Looman CW, Habbema JD, de Jong FH, et al. Serum antimullerian hormone levels best reflect the reproductive decline with age in normal women with proven fertility: A longitudinal study. Fertility and Sterility. 2005;**83**(4):979-987

[37] Fanchin R, Schonauer LM, Righini C, Frydman N, Frydman R, Taieb J. Serum anti-Müllerian hormone dynamics during controlled ovarian hyperstimulation. Human Reproduction. 2003;**18**:328-332

[38] Hehenkamp WJ, Looman CW, Themmen AP, de Jong FH, Te Velde ER, Broekmans FJ. Anti-Mullerian hormone levels in the spontaneous menstrual cycle do not show substantial fluctuation. The Journal of Clinical Endocrinology and Metabolism. 2006;**91**:4057-4063

[39] La Marca A, De Leo V, Giulini S, Orvieto R, Malmusi S, Giannella L, et al. Anti-Mullerian hormone in premenopausal women and after spontaneous or surgically induced menopause. Journal of the Society for Gynecologic Investigation. 2005;**12**:545-548

[40] La Marca A, Giulini S, Orvieto R, De Leo V, Volpe A. Anti-Mullerian hormone concentrations in maternal serum during pregnancy. Human Reproduction. 2005;**20**:1569-1572

[41] Somunkiran A, Yavuz T, Yucel O, Ozdemir I. Anti-Mullerian hormone levels during hormonal contraception in women with polycystic ovary syndrome. European Journal of Obstetrics, Gynecology, and Reproductive Biology. 2007;**134**:196-201

[42] La Marca A, Stabile G, Artenisio AC, Volpe A. Serum anti-Mullerian hormone throughout the human menstrual cycle. Human Reproduction. 2006;**21**:3103-3107

[43] Streuli I, Fraisse T, Pillet C, IbecheoleV, BischofP, deZieglerD. Serum antimullerian hormone levels remain stable throughout the menstrual cycle and after oral or vaginal administration of synthetic sex steroids. Fertility and Sterility. 2008;**90**:395-400

[44] Tsepelidis S, Devreker F, Demeestere I, Flahaut A, Gervy C, Englert Y. Stable serum levels of anti-Mullerian hormone during the menstrual cycle: A prospective study in normo-ovulatory women. Human Reproduction. 2007;**22**:1837-1840

[45] Plante BJ, Beamon C, Schmitt CL, Moldenhauer JS, Steiner AZ. Maternal antimullerian hormone levels do not predict fetal aneuploidy. Journal of Assisted Reproduction and Genetics. 2010;**27**:409-414

[46] Shim SH, Ha HI, Jung YW, Shim SS, Cho YK, Kim JY, et al. Maternal antimullerian hormone as a predictor of fetal aneuploidy occurring in an earlypregnancy loss. Obstetrics & Gynecology Science. 2015;**58**(6):494-500

[47] Fragouli E, Alfarawati S, Spath K, Jaroudi S, Sarasa J, Enciso M, et al. The origin and impact of embryonic aneuploidy. Human Genetics. 2013;**132**:1-13

[48] Handyside AH. Molecular origin of female meiotic aneuploidies. Biochimica et Biophysica Acta. 2012;**1822**:1913-1920

[49] Pellestor F, Andreo B, Anahory T, Hamamah S. The occurrence of aneuploidy in human: Lessons from the cytogenetic studies of human oocytes. European Journal of Medical Genetics. 2006;**49**:103-116

[50] Kuliev A, Zlatopolsky Z, Kirillova I, Spivakova J, Cieslak Janzen J. Meiosis errors in over 20,000 oocytes studied in the practice of preimplantation aneuploidy testing. Reproductive Biomedicine Online. 2011;**22**:2-8

[51] Battaglia DE, Goodwin P, Klein NA, Soules MR. Fertilization and early embryology: Influence of maternal age on meiotic spindle assembly oocytes from naturally cycling women. Human Reproduction. 1996;**11**:2217-2222

[52] Coticchio G, Guglielmo MC, Dal Canto M, Fadini R, Mignini Renzini M, De Ponti E, et al. Mechanistic foundations of the metaphase II spindle of human oocytes matured in vivo and in vitro. Human Reproduction. 2013;**28**:3271-3282

[53] Volarcik K, Sheean L, Goldfarb J, Woods L, Abdul-Karim FW, Hunt P. The meiotic competence of in-vitro matured human oocytes is influenced by donor age: Evidence that folliculogenesis is compromised in the reproductively aged ovary. Human Reproduction. 1998;**13**:154-160

[54] Angell RR. Predivision in human oocytes at meiosis-I—A mechanism for trisomy formation in man. Human Genetics. 1991;**86**:383-387

[55] Chiang T, Duncan FE, Schindler K, Schultz RM, Lampson MA. Evidence that weakened centromere cohesion is a leading cause of age-related aneuploidy in oocytes. Current Biology. 2010;**20**:1522-1528

[56] Yun Y, Lane SIR, Jones KT. Premature dyad separation in meiosis II is the major segregation error with maternal age in mouse oocytes. Development. 2014;**141**:199-208

[57] Duncan FE, Hornick JE, Lampson MA, Schultz RM, Shea LD, Woodruff TK. Chromosome cohesion decreases in human eggs with advanced maternal age. Aging Cell. 2012;**11**:1121-1124

[58] Allshire RC, Dempster M, Hastie ND. Human telomere contains at least three types of G-rich repeats distributed non-randomly. Nucleic Acids Research. 1989;**17**:4611-4627

[59] Shampay J, Blackburn EH. Generation of telomere-length heterogeneity in *Saccharomyces cerevisiae*. Proceedings of the National Academy of Sciences of the United States of America. 1988;**85**:534-538

[60] Aviv A. The epidemiology of human telomeres: Faults and promises. The Journals of Gerontology. Series A, Biological Sciences and Medical Sciences. 2008;**63**:979-983

[61] Aydos SE, Elhan AH, Tükün A. Is telomere length one of the determinants of reproductive life span? Archives of Gynecology and Obstetrics. 2005;**272**:113-116

[62] Keefe DL, Marquard K, Liu L. The telomere theory of reproductive senescence in women. Current Opinion in Obstetrics and Gynecology. 2006;**18**:280-285

[63] Betts DH, King WA. Telomerase activity and telomere detection during early bovine development. Developmental Genetics. 1999;**25**:397-403

[64] Eisenhauer KM, Gerstein RM, Chiu CP, Conti M, Hsueh AJ. Telomerase activity in female and male rat germ cells undergoing meiosis and in early embryos. Biology of Reproduction. 1997;**56**:1120-1125

[65] Kinugawa C, Murakami T, Okamura K, Yajima A. Telomerase activity in normal ovaries and premature ovarian failure. The Tohoku Journal of Experimental Medicine. 2000;**190**:231-238

[66] Liu JP, Li H. Telomerase in the ovary. Reproduction. 2010;**140**:215-222

[67] Herrera E, Samper E, Blasco MA. Telomere shortening in mTRK/K embryos is associated with failure to close the neural tube. EMBO Journal. 1999;**18**:1172-1181

[68] Lee HW, Blasco MA, Gottlieb GJ, Horner JW II, Greider CW, De Pinho RA. Essential role of mouse telomerase in highly proliferative organs. Nature. 1998;**392**:569-574

[69] Liu L, Blasco M, Trimarchi J, Keefe D. An essential role for functional telomeres in mouse germ cells during fertilization and early development. Developmental Biology. 2002;**249**:74-84

[70] Mania A, Mantzouratou A, Delhanty JD, Baio G, Serhal P, Sengupta SB. Telomere length in human blastocysts. Reproductive Biomedicine Online. 2014;**28**:624-637

[71] Plentz RR, Schlegelberger B, Flemming P, Gebel M, Kreipe H, Manns MP, et al. Telomere shortening correlates with increasing aneuploidy of chromosome 8 in human hepatocellular carcinoma. Hepatology. 2005;**42**:522-526

[72] Dorland M, van Montfrans JM, van Kooij RJ, Lambalk CB, te Velde ER. Normal telomere lengths in young mothers of children with Down's syndrome. Lancet. 1998;**352**:961-962

[73] Sabatier L, Ricoul M, Pottier G, Murnane JP. The loss of a single telomere can result in instability of multiple chromosomes in a human tumor cell line. Molecular Cancer Research. 2005;**3**:139-150

[74] Stewénius Y, Gorunova L, Jonson T, Larsson N, Höglund M, Mandahl N, et al. Structural and numerical chromosome changes in colon cancer develop through telomere-mediated anaphase bridges, not through mitotic multipolarity. Proceedings of the National Academy of Sciences of the United States of America. 2005;**102**:5541-5546

[75] Lin J, Smith DL, Blackburn EH. Mutant telomere sequences lead to impaired chromosome separation and a unique checkpoint response. Molecular Biology of the Cell. 2004;**15**(4):1623-1634

[76] van Noord PA, Dubas JS, Dorland M, Boersma H, te Velde E. Age at natural menopause in a population-based screening cohort: The role of menarche, fecundity, and lifestyle factors. Fertility and Sterility. 1997;**68**:95-102

[77] van Asselt KM, Kok HS. Age at menopause. A genetic epidemiological study [academic thesis]. The Netherlands: Utrecht; 2003

[78] Murabito JM, Yang Q, Fox C, Wilson PW, Cupples LA. Heritability of age at natural menopause in the Framingham Heart Study. The Journal of Clinical Endocrinology and Metabolism. 2005;**90**:3427-3430

[79] Torgerson DJ, Thomas RE, Reid DM. Mothers and daughters menopausal ages: Is there a link? European Journal of Obstetrics, Gynecology, and Reproductive Biology. 1997;**74**:63-66

[80] van Asselt KM, Kok HS, Pearson PL, Dubas JS, Peeters PH, Te Velde ER, et al. Heritability of menopausal age in mothers and daughters. Fertility and Sterility. 2004;**82**:1348-1351

[81] Laissue P, Vinci G, Veitia RA, Fellous M. Recent advances in the study of genes involved in non-syndromic premature ovarian failure. Molecular and Cellular Endocrinology. 2008;**282**:101-111

[82] Laissue P, Lakhal B, Benayoun BA, Dipietromaria A, Braham R, Elghezal H, et al. Functional evidence implicating FOXL2 in non syndromic premature ovarian failure and in the regulation of the transcription factor OSR2. Journal of Medical Genetics. 2009;**46**(7):455-457

[83] Kok HS, van Asselt KM, van der Schouw YT, Peeters PH, Wijmenga C. Genetic studies to identify genes underlying menopausal age. Human Reproduction Update. 2005;**11**:483-493

[84] Skillern A, Rajkovic A. Recent developments in identifying genetic determinants of premature ovarian failure. Sexual Development. 2008;**2**:228-243

[85] Knauff EA, Wijmenga C, van't Slot R, Franke L, Fauser BC. Genome wide high density SNP-CGH reveals several new deletion copy number variants on the X chromosome in POF patients. Reproductive Sciences. 2009;**15**:601

[86] McCarroll SA. Extending genome-wide association studies to copy-number variation. Human Molecular Genetics. 2008;**17**:R135-R142

[87] Rodriguez-Revenga L, Mila M, Rosenberg C, Lamb A, Lee C. Structural variation in the human genome: The impact of copy number variants on clinical diagnosis. Genetics in Medicine. 2007;**9**:600-606

[88] Wang K, Li M, Hadley D, Liu R, Glessner J, Grant SF, et al. Penn CNV: An integrated hidden Markov model designed for high-resolution copy number variation detection in whole-genome SNP genotyping data. Genome Research. 2007;**17**:1665-1674

[89] Di Pasquale E, Rossetti R, Marozzi A, Bodega B, Borgato S, Cavallo L, et al. Identification of new variants of human BMP15 gene in a large cohort of women with premature ovarian failure. The Journal of Clinical Endocrinology and Metabolism. 2006;**91**:1976-1979

[90] Dixit H, Rao LK, Padmalatha VV, Kanakavalli M, Deenadayal M, Gupta N, et al. Missense mutations in the BMP15 gene are associated with ovarian failure. Human Genetics. 2006;**119**:408-415

[91] Laissue P, Christin-Maitre S, Touraine P, Kuttenn F, Ritvos O, Aittomaki K, et al. Mutations and sequence variants in GDF9 and BMP15 in patients with premature ovarian failure. European Journal of Endocrinology. 2006;**154**:739-744

[92] Schmidt D, Ovitt CE, Anlag K, Fehsenfeld S, Gredsted L, Treier AC, et al. The murine winged-helix transcription factor Foxl2 is required for granulosa cell

differentiation and ovary maintenance. Development. 2004;**131**:933-942

[93] Kok HS, van Asselt KM, van der Schouw YT, van der Tweel I, Peeters PH, Wilson PW, et al. Heart disease risk determines menopausal age rather than the reverse. Journal of the American College of Cardiology. 2006;**47**:1976-1983

[94] Koochmeshgi J, Hosseini-Mazinani SM, Morteza Seifati S, Hosein-Pur-Nobari N, Teimoori-Toolabi L. Apolipoprotein E genotype and age at menopause. Annals of the New York Academy of Sciences. 2004;**1019**:564-567

[95] Pripp U, Eriksson-Berg M, Orth-Gome'r K, Schenck-Gustafsson K, Landgren BM. Does body mass index, smoking, lipoprotein levels, surgically induced menopause, hormone replacement therapy, years since menopause, or age affect hemostasis in postmenopausal women? Gender Medicine. 2005;**2**:88-95

[96] Huber A, Grimm C, Huber JC, Schneeberger C, Leodolter S, Reinthaller A, et al. A common polymorphism within the steroid 5-α-reductase type 2 gene and timing of menopause in Caucasian women. European Journal of Obstetrics, Gynecology, and Reproductive Biology. 2006;**125**:221-225

[97] Hefler LA, Grimm C, Heinze G, Schneeberger C, Mueller MW, MuendleinA,etal.Estrogen-metabolizing gene polymorphisms and age at natural menopause in Caucasian women. Human Reproduction. 2005;**20**:1422-1427

[98] Weel AE, Uitterlinden AG, Westendorp IC, Burger H, Schuit SC, Hofman A, et al. Estrogen receptor polymorphism predicts the onset of natural and surgical menopause. The Journal of Clinical Endocrinology and Metabolism. 1999;**84**:3146-3150

[99] Hou N, Chen S, Chen F, Jiang M, Zhang J, Yang Y, et al. Association between premature ovarian failure, polymorphisms in MTHFR and MTRRgenes and serum homocysteine concentration. Reproductive Biomedicine Online. 2016;**32**(4):407-413

[100] Rah H, Jeon YJ, Choi Y, Shim SH, Yoon TK, Choi DH, et al. Association of methylenetetrahydrofolate reductase (MTHFR 677C>T) and thymidylatesynthase (TSER and TS 1494del6) polymorphisms with premature ovarian failure in Korean women. Menopause. 2012;**19**(11):1260-1266

[101] Dutta S, Das AB, Mukhopadhyay K. Risk of Down syndrome conferred by MTHFR C677T polymorphism: Ethnic variations. Indian Journal of Human Genetics. 2007;**13**(2):76-77

[102] James SJ, Pogribna M, Pofribny IP, Melnyk S, Hine RJ, Gibson JB, et al. Abnormal folate metaboloism and mutation in the methylenetetrahydrofolate reductase gene may be maternal risk factors for Down syndrome. American Journal of Clinical Nutrition. 1999;**70**:495-501

[103] Martínez-Frías ML, Bermejo E, Rodríguez-Pinilla E, Prieto D, Prieto L. MTHFR 677C-T polymorphism is not excluded as maternal risk for Down syndrome among Turkish women. American Journal of Medical Genetics. Part A. 2005;**134**(4):461-462

[104] Meguid NA, Dardir AA, Khass M, Hossieny LE, Ezzat A, El Awady MK. MTHFR genetic polymorphism as a risk factor in Egyptian mothers with Down syndrome children. Disease Markers. 2008;**24**(1):19-26

[105] He C, Kraft P, Chen C, Buring JE, Pare G, Hankinson SE, et al. Genome-wide association studies identify loci associated with age at menarche and age at natural menopause. Nature Genetics. 2009;**41**:724-728

[106] Stolk L, Zhai G, van Meurs JB, Verbiest MM, Visser JA, Estrada K, et al. Loci at chromosomes 13, 19 and 20 influence age at natural menopause. Nature Genetics. 2009;**41**:645-647

[107] Penrose LS. The relative effect of paternal and maternal age in mongolism. Journal of Genetics. 1933;**27**:219-224

[108] Chiang T, Schultz RM, Lampson MA. Age-dependent susceptibility of chromosomecohesion to premature separase activation in mouse oocytes. Biology of Reproduction. 2011;**85**(6):1279-1283. DOI: 10.1095/biolreprod.111.094094. Epub 2011 Aug 24. PubMedPMID: 21865557; PubMed Central PMCID: PMC3223255

[109] Kitajima TS, Sakuno T, Ishiguro K, Iemura S, Natsume T, Kawashima SA, et al. Shugoshin collaborates with protein phosphatase 2A to protect cohesin. Nature. 2006;**441**(7089):46-52. Epub 2006 Mar 15. PubMed PMID: 16541025

[110] Riedel CG, Katis VL, Katou Y, Mori S, Itoh T, Helmhart W, et al. Protein phosphatase 2A protects centromeric sister chromatid cohesion during meiosis I. Nature. 2006;**441**(7089):53-61. Epub 2006 Mar 15. PubMed PMID: 16541024

[111] Hodges CA, Revenkova E, Jessberger R, Hassold TJ, Hunt PA. SMC1beta-deficientfemale mice provide evidence that cohesins are a missing link in age-related nondisjunction. Nature Genetics. 2005;**37**(12):1351-1355. Epub 2005 Oct 30. PubMed PMID: 16258540

[112] Miyazaki WY, Orr Weaver TL. Sister chromatid misbehavior in Drosophila ord mutants. Genetics. 1992;**132**(1047):1061. PMID: 1459426

[113] Gilliland WD, Hawley RS. Cohesin and the maternal age effect. Cell. 2005;**123**(3):371-373. PubMed PMID: 16269329

[114] Pan H, Ma P, Zhu W, Schultz RM. Age-associated increase in aneuploidy and changes in gene expression in mouse eggs. Developmental Biology. 2008;**316**(2):397-407. DOI: 10.1016/j.ydbio.2008.01.048. Epub 2008 Feb 15. PubMed PMID: 18342300; PubMed Central PMCID: PMC2374949

[115] Brunet S, Pahlavan G, Taylor S, Maro B. Functionality of the spindle checkpoint during the first meiotic division of mammalian oocytes. Reproduction. 2003;**126**:443-450

[116] Hached K, Xie SZ, Buffin E, Cladiere D, Rachez C, Sacras M, et al. Mps1 at kinetochores is essential for female mouse meiosis I. Development. 2011;**138**:2261-2271

[117] Lane SI, Chang HY, Jennings PC, Jones KT. The Aurora kinase inhibitorZM447439 accelerates first meiosis in mouse oocytes by overriding the spindle assembly checkpoint. Reproduction. 2010;**140**:521-530

[118] Niault T, Hached K, Sotillo R, Sorger PK, Maro B, Benezra R, et al. Changing Mad2 levels affects chromosome segregation and spindle assembly checkpoint control in female mouse meiosis I. PLoS One. 2007;**e1165**:2

[119] Wassmann K, Niault T, Maro B. Metaphase I arrest upon activation of the Mad2-dependent spindle checkpoint in mouse oocytes. Current Biology. 2003;**13**:1596-1608

[120] Duncan FE, Chiang T, Schultz RM, Lampson MA. Evidence that adefective spindle assembly checkpoint is not the primary cause of maternalage-associated aneuploidy in mouse eggs. Biology of Reproduction. 2009;**81**:768-776

[121] Eichenlaub-Ritter U, Staubach N, Trapphoff T. Chromosomal and cytoplasmic context determines predisposition to maternal age-related aneuploidy: Brief overview and update on MCAK in mammalian oocytes. Biochemical Society Transactions. 2010;**38**(6):1681-1686. DOI: 10.1042/BST0381681. PubMed PMID: 21118147

[122] Gougeon A, Ecochard R, Thalabard JC. Age-related changes of the population of human ovarian follicles: Increase in the disappearance rate of non-growing andearly-growing follicles in aging women. Biology of Reproduction. 1994;**50**(3):653-663. PubMed PMID: 8167237

[123] Gougeon A. Ovarian follicular growth in humans: Ovarian ageing and population of growing follicles. Maturitas. 1998;**30**(2):137-142. Review. PubMed PMID: 9871908

[124] Hansen KR, Knowlton NS, Thyer AC, Charleston JS, Soules MR, Klein NA. A newmodel of reproductive aging: The decline in ovarian non-growing follicle number from birth to menopause. Human Reproduction. 2008;**23**(3):699-708. doi: 10.1093/humrep/dem408. Epub 2008 Jan 11. PubMed PMID: 18192670

[125] Warren AC, Chakravarti A, Wong C, Slaugenhaupt SA, Halloran SL, Watkins PC, et al. Evidence for reduced recombination on the nondisjoined chromosomes 21 in Down syndrome. Science. 1987;**237**:652-654

[126] Carpenter AT. Chiasma function. Cell. 1994;**77**:957-962

[127] Koehler KE, Hawley RS, Sherman S, Hassold T. Recombination and nondisjunctionin humans and flies. Human Molecular Genetics. 1996;**5**:1495-1504

[128] Moore DP, Miyazaki WY, Tomkiel JE, Orr-Weaver TL. Double or nothing: A *Drosophila* mutation affecting meiotic chromosome segregation in both females and males. Genetics. 1994;**136**:953-964

[129] Rasooly RS, New CM, Zhang P, Hawley RS, Baker BS. The lethal(1) TW-6cs mutationof *Drosophila melanogaster* is a dominant antimorphic allele of nod and is associated with a single base change in the putative ATP-binding domain. Genetics. 1991;**129**:409-422

[130] Krawchuk MD, Wahls WP. Centromere mapping functions for aneuploid meioticproducts: Analysis of rec8, rec10 and rec11 mutants of the fission yeast *Schizosaccharomyces pombe*. Genetics. 1999;**153**:49-55

[131] Sears DD, Hegemann JH, Shero JH, Hieter P. Cis-acting determinants affectingcentromere function, sister-chromatid cohesion and reciprocal recombinationduring meiosis in *Saccharomyces cerevisiae*. Genetics. 1995;**139**:1159-1173

[132] Zetka MC, Rose AM. Mutant rec-1 eliminates the meiotic pattern of crossing over in *Caenorhabditis elegans*. Genetics. 1995;**141**:1339-1349

[133] Lamb NE, Sherman SL, Hassold TJ. Effect of meiotic recombination on theproduction of aneuploid gametes in humans. Cytogenetic and Genome Research. 2005;**111**:250-255

[134] Ghosh S, Feingold E, Dey SK. Etiology of Down syndrome: Evidence for consistent association among altered meiotic recombination, nondisjunction

and maternal age across populations. American Journal of Medical Genetics. 2009;**149A**:1415-1420

[135] Sherman SL, Petersen MB, Freeman SB, Hersey J, Pettay D, Taft L, et al. Non-disjunction of chromosome 21 in maternal meiosis I: Evidence for a maternal age-dependent mechanism involving reducedrecombination. Human Molecular Genetics. 1994;**3**:1529-1535

[136] Bugge M, Collins A, Petersen MB, Fisher J, Brandt C, Hertz JM, et al. Non-disjunction of chromosome 18. Human Molecular Genetics. 1998;**7**:661-669

[137] Robinson WP, Kuchinka BD, Bernasconi F, Petersen MB, Schulze A, Brondum-Nielsen K, et al. Maternal meiosis I non-disjunction ofchromosome 15: Dependence of the maternal age effect on level of recombination. Human Molecular Genetics. 1998;**7**:1011-1019

[138] Thomas NS, Ennis S, Sharp AJ, Durkie M, Hassold TJ, Collins AR, et al. Maternalsex chromosome non-disjunction: Evidence for X chromosome-specific risk factors. Human Molecular Genetics. 2001;**10**:243-250

Chapter 4

Gene Polymorphisms That Predispose Women for Down Syndrome Child Birth

Sujay Ghosh and Papiya Ghosh

Abstract

Down syndrome caused by presence of extra chromosome 21 originates from nondisjunction during parental gametogenesis. For overwhelming cases, the error occurs in oocyte and all the nondisjunction events are not stochastic. With increasing number of research efforts, it has come to know that maternal genetic architecture may be considered as risk factors for chromosomal errors. Polymorphisms of the genes involved in chromosome segregation, recombination and folic acid metabolisms have been investigated for their association with Down syndrome child birth. But the results are conflicting owing to ethnic and sociocultural differences. Here, we have discussed and summarized the outcome of the studies conducted on different population sample from different parts of world and tried to figure out the common polymorphisms, which could be used as makers for preconceptional screening of Down syndrome child birth risk among the women.

Keywords: down syndrome, maternal genotype, polymorphism, meiotic nondisjunction

1. Introduction

Down syndrome (DS), the most common form of live born intellectual disability in human is caused by trisomy condition of chromosome 21 (Ch21). The trisomy 21 condition arise from nonseparation or nondisjunction (NDJ) of Ch21 in germinal cells that leads to production of disomic gamete which upon fertilization with gamete with correct chromosome count from opposite sex produces trisomic zygote. For overwhelming majority of cases, the error arises in oocyte and this may be due to protracted phase of oocyte development. The lengthy process of oocyte maturation that includes two halts, one at meiotic I diplotene and another before the entry in second meiotic division, provides opportunity to environmental insults to accumulate in ovarian microenvironment that may perturb the process of chromosome segregation.

The first identified risk factor for Down syndrome birth is advanced maternal age of conception. It was identified that [1], women of age 32 years and above have higher risk of having Down syndrome baby. Subsequently, with the help of polymorphic variants of short tandem repeat (STR) makers on Ch21 scientists have characterized that recombination error may be the molecular risk factors for Ch21 NDJ. With elaborate analyses, considering both the maternal age and pattern of recombination, the US researcher group [2] and Indian researcher group [3] have characterized the interaction between maternal age and erroneous pattern of recombination on non-disjoined chromosome. No chiasma formation or single telomeric chiasma have been proved as risk of Ch21NDJ at MI among the younger mothers (age < 29 years). On contrary, single centromeric chiasma has been identified as risk factors for MII errors among the older women (age > 34 years).

With subsequent analyses of maternal molecular age, it has been proved that mothers of Down syndrome baby have shorter average telomere length than do the mothers of same chronological age and have euploid healthy baby [4, 5]. The authors proposed that a group of women may suffer from advanced molecular and genetic aging and intuitively carry predisposition for NDJ. It is really difficult to interpret whether NDJ is the result of rapid shortening of telomere or telomere shortening and NDJ are linked by some common risk factors, instead it can be said pleiotrophic effects of some genes may relate maternal aging with risk of NDJ. Moreover, frequent occurrence Ch21 NDJ among younger women reinforces the intuitive idea of genetic predisposition for Ch21 NDJ where advancing maternal age is not an issue.

As far as published literatures are concerned studies for identifying the genetic predisposition for DS child birth among the women are not sufficient. Very few initiatives in this regard have been recorded. Of them the recombination regulator genes and folate metabolism regulator genes are major. So, this chapter presents recent updates on finding of the gene polymorphisms that exhibited significant association with Down syndrome birth.

2. PR/SET domain 9 (PRDM9)

The gene is located on chromosome 5 (5p14.2). The protein coded by this gene is a zinc finger protein with histone methyltransferase activity that catalyzes trimethylation of histone H3 lysine 4 (H3K4me3) during meiotic prophase. This protein contains multiple domains, including a Kruppel-associated box (KRAB) domain, an SSX repression domain (SSXRD), a PRD1-BF1 and RIZ homologous region, a subclass of SET (PR/SET) domain, and a tandem array of C2H2 zinc fingers. The zinc finger array recognizes a short sequence motif of histone, leading to local H3K4me3, and meiotic recombination hotspot activity.

Experimental deletion of the gene in mice leads to the production of gametes blocked at pachytene of meiosis I that show a reduced number of Dmc1 loci, a protein that indicates the sites of meiotic crossovers [6]. The major allele A of PRDM9 binds a 13 bp DNA motif enriched at recombination hot spot, namely, CNCCNTNNCCNC [7]. Further, allelic variation in the zinc finger motif of PRDM9 exhibited association with differential hotspot usage in human recombination [8]. Carriers of PRDM9 minor alleles display reduced recombination at meiotic hotspots [8]. All these preceding observation led to the study [9] to inquire whether PRDM9 variants exhibit association with the recombination variation that underlies the NDJ events.

In this study [9] by US researcher group included 235 mothers having DS child and 85 controls having euploid baby. For characterizing the recombination profile along the 21q, the authors used genotyping with 1536 SNP loci on 21q by the Illumina Golden Gate Assay. The authors scored for 17% of cases of MI error without any recombination events carry homozygosity of minor alleles in contrast to only 2% of MI with single exchange category. The logistic regression analyses revealed women from MI without any exchange category are 2.45 times more likely to have risk of NDJ and Down syndrome birth than do the controls when carry at least one minor allele in heterozygous condition. The authors found less affinity of minor allele of ZF motif of PRDM9 and they tried to justify this reduced binding of PRDM9 to the recombination hotspot may cause lack of recombination events on 21q and NDJ of Ch21. This notion needs further confirmation by other studies on different DS populations of ethnic variations for considering as acceptable hypothesis.

3. Apolipoprotein E (APOE)

This gene is located on chromosome 19 (19q13.32) and encodes a protein which is essential for normal catabolism of triglyceride-rich lipoprotein. It binds to specific receptor on hepatocytes and peripheral cell receptors. Mutations in this gene leads to familial dysbetalipoproteinemia, or type III hyperlipoproteinemia (HLP III), which is characterized by increased plasma cholesterol and triglycerides due of impaired clearance of chylomicron and VLDL remnants. The gene is expressed specifically in liver, kidney, adipose, adrenal, spleen and neuronal tissues along with some other organs at low level.

Initial study that addressed the maternal APOE genotypes as risk factors of DS birth [10] reported presence of APOE4 allele among women may predispose them for MII NDJ at the younger age, but not at older age. The authors observed in young mothers with a meiosis II error, epsilon4 frequency was 30.0%, which was significantly higher than in older mothers with a meiosis II error (13.0%, $P = 0.03$).

But the study [11] conducted on Spanish population reported some opposite trend. The authors have observed an increased frequency of APOE4 allele among MI mother of age < 28 years as compared to MI mothers of age > 28 years. But this study did not confirm any association of maternal APOE4 genotype with MII error. The study on Colombian population [12] has revealed preferential occurrence of APOE4 allele in DS and their parents (11%) than among the controls (9%) though the difference was found insignificant statistically. More studies are needed to confirm the association between APOE4 allele in maternal genome and Ch21 NDJ.

4. Presenilin I (PSEN1)

This gene is located at the position 14q24.2 and known for its pleiotrophic effects. It has many isoforms that perform variety of functions. The polymorphisms of this gene were first reported for its association with Alzheimer disease. Later, it was tested for risk assessment in women having DS child.

As far as published literatures are concerned, only two studies have been conducted on PSEN 1 polymorphisms as a maternal risk factor for DS birth. The initial study was done on US population [13] where the authors find an association between a polymorphism in intron 8 of maternal genotype with DS birth. This study included168 probands with free trisomy 21 and recorded an increased frequency of allele 1 in mothers with a meiosis II error (70.8%) than among the mothers of meiosis I error (52.7%, $P < 0.01$), with an excess of the 11 genotype in the meiosis II mothers. Moreover, the author tested polymorphic variants of APOE gene and found the frequency of allele 1 in mothers carrying APOE4 allele (68.0%) was higher than in mothers without APOE4 (52.2%, $P < 0.01$). The author hypothesizes that the PSEN-1 intronic polymorphism might be involved in chromosomal nondisjunction through an influence on the expression level of PS-1 or due to linkage disequilibrium with biologically relevant polymorphisms in or outside the PS-1 gene.

Similar study was conducted on a population samples from India [14]. In this study, 170 Down syndrome patients, grouped according to maternal meiotic stage of NDJ and maternal age at conception, and their parents were genotyped for PSEN-1 intron-8 and APOE polymorphisms. The estimated frequencies of the PSEN-1 T allele and TT genotype, in the presence of the APOE4 allele, were significantly higher among young mothers (< 35 years) with meiosis II NDJ than in young control mothers (96.43 vs. 65.91% P = 0.0002 and 92.86 vs. 45.45% P < 0.0001, respectively) but not among mothers with meiosis I NDJ. The author hypothesized that the co-occurrence of the PSEN-1 T allele and the APOE 4 allele synergistically increases the risk of meiotic segregation error II among young.

5. Methylenetetrahydrofolate reductase (MTHFR)

This gene is located at 1p36.22 and the 12 exon long reading frame encodes an enzyme that catalyzes the reduction of 5,10-methylene tetra hydro folate to 5-methyl tetra hydro folate, which is required for the remethylation of homocysteine to methionine. A common MTHFR 677C > T polymorphism (rs1801133) that results in Ala222Val amino acid substitution, is responsible for reduced enzyme activity. The homozygous TT genotype causes dimer destabilization under conditions of reduced folate availability [15, 16]. It was reported initially [17] in the year 1999, that increased plasma hcy level and an increased frequency of both MTHFR 677CT and TT genotypes among the mothers of DS individuals are strongly linked and since then this polymorphism has been tested in more than 30 case-control studies across the globe and confirmed this association with very few exceptions. As far as published literatures are concerned five large meta-analyses have been done till date between the year 2013 and 2014 to address this issue [18–22], with the latest one that includes data from 34 case-control studies for a total of 3.098 women having DS child and 4.852 control mothers [21]. The outcome of all these meta-analyses suggest that the overall risk as represented by odds ratio (OR), for the birth of a child with Trisomy21 to the women who are carriers of the 677 T allele ranges from 1.2 to 1.5 according to the various genetic models under investigation, i.e., allele contrast, dominant, recessive, co-dominant, etc. Subsequent data stratification into ethnic groups revealed that the risk is higher in Asians (OR = 1.5), and lower in Caucasians and/or other groups (OR usually ranging between 1.0 and 1.4) [19, 20, 22]. The meta-analyses performed by Wu et al. [19]; Yang et al. [20]; Rai et al. [21]; Victorino et al. [22] revealed that the frequency of the MTHFR 677 T allele is higher in Caucasian mother of DS child (ranging from 35.6 to 41.5%), followed by Brazilians (ranging from 33.5 to 33.9%), and lower in Asian populations (ranging from 20.0 to 32.3%). When epidemiological data were stratified according to the geographic origin of the mothers and found that the higher risk in Asians (OR = 1.53; 95% CI = 1.29–1.82), followed by Americans (OR = 1.23; 95% CI = 1.07–1.39), and the association remain insignificant for Europeans (OR = 1.04; 95% CI = 0.93–1.16) [21]. When the data was stratified according to latitude, exhibited a significant association of the MTHFR 677C > T polymorphism with DS birth insub-tropical populations (both TT vs. CC and CT vs. CC carriers), followed by tropical regions (only CT vs. CC carriers), but no significant effect was evident in the population from northern temperate region of the globe. These observations suggest complex gene–environment interactions, which might be a product of differences in allele frequencies among different populations in association with different nutritional status and exposure to environmental factors, such as solar radiation, that could interfere with folate bioavailability [16, 18, 22, 23]. Interestingly, scientists have observed association of the MTHFR 677C > T polymorphism with both chromosome 13 and 21 malsegregation events in lymphocytes from the mothers of DS child [23, 24].

Another common MTHFR polymorphism, the MTHFR 1298A > C one (rs1801131), causes Glu429Ala aminoacidic change. Meta-analysis revealed that the frequency of the MTHFR minor 1298C allele is higher in Asians (~40.0%), with little less frequency among Caucasians (~35.0%) and Brazilians (upto 25.0%) [22]. Interestingly, no studies have demonstrated MTHFR 1298A > C polymorphism is an independent maternal risk factor for the birth of a child with DS. Instead, However, case-control studies demonstrated that genotypes that carry both the MTHFR 677C > T and 1298A > C polymorphisms increase the maternal risk synergistically for a birth of a child with trisomy 21 more than the presence of the single polymorphic site MTHFR 677C > T one alone. These observations suggest intuitive functional interaction of both polymorphisms on protein stability and activity [25–29]. The maternal double homozygous 677TT-1298CC genotype leads to MTHFR protein instability and inactivity, often resulting in prenatal death [16].

6. Methionine synthase and methionine synthase reductase (*MTR* and *MTRR*)

The gene named as 5-methyltetrahydrofolate-homocysteine methyltransferase (MTR) or methionine synthase in short is located at 1q43 and carries 33 exons. It is a cobalamin-dependent enzyme that catalyzes the transmethylation of homocystein to methionine and MTRR, which is a NADPH-dependent diflavin enzyme, needed for activation of MTR. On the other hand the gene5-methyltetrahydrofolate-homocysteine methyltransferase reductase of MTRR is located at 5p15.31 in human genome. This protein functions in the synthesis of methionine by regenerating methionine synthase (MTR) to a functional state.

The second polymorphism of the gene *MTRR* that exhibited association with DS birth among North American women is rs1801394; 66A > G substitution which causes Ile22Met amino acid change [30]. Subsequent studies on different population samples provide conflicting results. Nevertheless, the meta-analysis conducted in 2009 on 623 DS bearing and 936 control mothers [31], confirmed association of this polymorphism in maternal genome with the elevated risk of having DS baby. Further analyses with stratified data, performed in recent time [32, 33], suggest a significant effect in Caucasians under both dominant and recessive genetic models. The estimated score for minor Allele "G" among Caucasian women was 35.8–54.3%, among Brazilian women was from 40.0 to 48.0% and among Asian mothers was from 41.5 to 62.5% [32–34]. Furthermore, when Caucasian samples were stratified by geographic and demographic criteria the estimates revealed that the risk is higher in those of non-residential European descent (OR = 1.47; 95% CI = 1.02–2.11; dominant model) than in residential European Caucasians (OR = 1.31; 95% CI = 1.01–1.70; dominant model). On contrary, when the study was conducted on the Caucasian from Mediterranean regions no significant association was observed (OR = 1.19; 95% CI = 0.91–1.55; dominant model), which suggests that the manifestation of the effect of MTRR rs1801394 66A > G is also dependent on geographic and dietary factors [33].

Recently, another *MTRR* polymorphism, namely *MTRR* 524C > T (rs1532268) that causes Ser175Leu replacement in peptide chain, has been identified as related to the maternal risk of birth of a child with DS [35] among Chinese women. This study reported decreased maternal risk for carriers of the 524 T allele that was associated with reduced hcy levels in Chinese women. But the study did not address the issue of but did not analyze the linkage or interaction of *MTRR* 524C > T (rs1532268) with the *MTRR* 66A > G sites [35].

As far as published literatures on the MTR gene polymorphisms are concerned, the *MTR* 2756A > G polymorphism (rs1805087) in maternal genome, leading to the Asp919Gly substitution, was the third variant of the folate pathway to be associated with DS birth [36]. However, subsequent case-control studies failed to confirm this association, and recent meta-analyses confirmed that the *MTR* 2756A > G polymorphism is not an independent maternal risk factor for DS birth [20, 32, 37], rather a strong relation with *MTRR* 66A > G has been evident. The estimated frequency of minor allele 'G' of this polymorphic site in the European and mixed Brazilian populations of women having DS child is 18–21% [37], while the estimate is less than 10% in the Asian women [38]. A large cohort study on Italian population samples [33, 37], revealed the *MTRR* 66A > G polymorphism, but not the *MTR* 2756A > G one, was associated with increased serum folate levels among the GG carriers women. On the other hand study on Brazilian population has [29] reported association of *MTRR* AG and GG genotypes with high methylmalonic acid (MMA) concentrations, an indicator of the vitamin B12 status. However, when both the polymorphisms *MTR* 2756AA/*MTRR* 66GG were present in women having DS child exhibited association with increased serum folate levels, while the carriers of the *MTR* 2756GG/*MTRR* 66AA genotype exhibited reduced folate and hcy levels [33]. Such combined presence of *MTHFR/MTRR* or *MTRR/MTR* genotypes among the mother of DS, has been many reported by many authors who worked on different ethnic population samples [23, 33, 34, 36, 38, 39].

7. Reduced folate carrier (*RFC1 or SLC19A1*)

The gene is actually named ***solute carrier family 19 member 1***, located at 21q22.3 and carries 17 exons. The protein expresses ubiquitously and is the major transport system in mammalian tissues for folate cofactors and regulates intracellular concentration of folate [40]. Though not universal, some workers have reported risk association with polymorphic allele in maternal genome with DS birth. The polymorphic variation *RFC1* 80G > A polymorphism (rs1051266), causes Arg27His replacement in protein chain. This polymorphic sites exhibited association with increased plasma hcy levels in homozygous GG genotype when present together with *MTHFR* 677TT [41] homozygous variants. Similarly study on Italian population [42] observed a borderline significant association of maternal genotype *RFC1* 80GG/*MTHFR* 677TT and DS birth and protective negative association with *RFC1* 80(AA or AG)/*MTHFR* 1298AA genotypes. Two recent meta-analyses [20, 33] suggest that the polymorphism *RFC1* 80G > A is independent maternal risk factor for DS birth with ORs ranging from 1.1 to 1.3. When stratified analyses has been conducted, the*RFC1* 80G allele exhibited higher frequency in Caucasian and Brazilian women having DS child (ranging between 49.0 and 54.0%) than in Asian ones (36.0–36.5%) [33]. Further population based studies are needed to confirm the implication of this polymorphism as a maternal risk factor for DS birth.

8. Cystathionine β-synthase (*CBS*)

The gene is located on chromsome21 at 21q22.3 and encodes a hemoprotein that catalyzes the condensation of hcy and serine to form cystathionine in the transsulfuration pathway. This enzyme is activated by adenosyl methionine and pyridoxal phosphate acts as co-factor in this reaction. So far published literatures are concerned two common polymorphisms have been studied as maternal risk factors for DS birth. One of them is an insertion of 68-bp within exon 8 that results in the duplication of a splice site at the intron7/exon 8 junction of the gene [43]. Very recent meta-analyses, performed with 825 mothers of DS child and 1.034 control did not find association of the *CBS* 844ins68 allele and maternal risk of having a DS child [20, 32]. The second polymorphic variants is an 833 T > C substitution (rs5742905) that causes missense mutationIle278Thr associated with mild hyperhomocysteinemia [44]. Results of association studies related to this site are contradictory and non-conclusive [29, 35], so further study is warrant to reveal its implication in DS birth.

9. Methylenetetrahydrofolate dehydrogenase (*MTHFD1*)

The genetic position of this gene is 14q23.3 and three distinct enzymatic activities, 5,10-methylenetetrahydrofolate-dehydrogenase,-5,10-methenyltetrahydrofolate-cyclohydrolase and 10-formyltetrahydrofolate synthetase. Each of these activities catalyzes one of the three sequential reactions in the interconversion of 1-carbon derivatives of tetrahydrofolate. The *MTHFD1* 1958G > A polymorphism (rs2236225), that causes missense change Arg653Gln which in turn reduces enzyme stability and activity and was first identified maternal genetic risk factor for trisomy 21 in Southern Italian women, exhibited association with DS risk in combination-with-the *RFC1* 80G > A-polymorphism-(the combined *MTHFD1* 1958AA/*RFC1*80GG genotype) [27]. The results of subsequent studies on other population were contradictory [29, 38, 45, 46]. Very recent meta-analysis [32] that included 497 mothers of Ds child and 930 controls, revealed a weak association with maternal heterozygous GA genotype than GG homozygous carriers (OR = 1.33; 95% CI = 1.01–1.75). The result of this single study may not sufficient to draw any inference and more study on other populations is warrant.

10. Transcobalamin (*TCN2*)

The gene is located on chromosome 22 at 22q12.2. This protein can bind cobalamin and helps in its cellular uptake by specific membrane receptors (TCR). The study of this gene for its association with DS birth is limited. A common variant *TCN2* 776C > G (rs1801198), that results in Arg232Pro replacement and impairs cobalamin metabolism [47] exhibited association with maternal risk of DS birth either alone [29], or in combination with *MTR* or MTHFR variants. The genotype *TCN2* 776CC/*MTR* 2756AG-[48]-or *TCN2* 776CG/*MTHFR* 677TT [38] have shown association with DS birth. But recent meta-analysis [32] did not confirm this association. The second polymorphism of that gene namely *TCN2* 67A > G (rs9606756) that causes Ile23Val substitution has been studied only in Brazilian population and did not find any association with maternal risk for a DS birth [29].

11. DNA methyltransferase 3B (*DNMT3B*)

This gene is located on chromosome 20 at 20q11.21 and encodes a de novo DNA methyl transferase. The enzyme is located primarily in nucleus and developmentally regulated. Two recent independent studies one on Italian and another on Indian population suggested the polymorphisms of DNMT3B might be associated with DS birth as maternal risk factors. In the study on Italian population [37] the authors genotyped 172 mothers with DS and 157 control mothers and found a decreased risk of birth of a child with DS among the mother who are carrier of DNMT3B 579G > T (rs1569686) minor allele T. Further, the author suggested that the combined *DNMT3B*-579GT/-149CC genotype was associated with an even more reduced maternal risk of birth of DS. That means the said genotypes have some protective implication on chromosome 21 NDJ. In Indian study [49] the author tested 150 mothers with Down syndrome and 172 control and found no significant difference in allelic and genotype frequency for individual loci between cases and controls, but found a significant difference in the frequency of haplotype rs1569686 -579G: rs2424913 -149 T which exhibited preferential occurrence among the DS child bearing mothers. Further study is needed to validate this association.

12. Serine-hydroxymethyltransferase (*SHMT*), thymidylate synthase (*TYMS*), and dihydrofolate reductase (*DHFR*)

The gene ***SHMT***TYMS and ***DHFR*** are located at 17p11.2, 18p11.32 and 5q14.1 respectively. SHMT coverts tetrahydrofolate (THF) into 5,10-methyleneTHF using serine as the one-carbon donor. This THF is then used for thymidylate synthesis in the reaction catalyzed by TYMS that produces dTMP and dihydrofolate (DHF). DHF is then reduced back to THF by DHFR. As far published literatures are concerned the polymorphisms of *SHMT, TYMS*, and *DHFR* have been analyzed as maternal risk factors for DS birth only in one case-control study each [50–52]. The *SHMT*1420C > T polymorphism (rs1979277), which causes Leu474Phe replacement and defects in nuclear transport of SHMT, was investigated [53] in 105 DS bearing and 185 control mothers from Brazil, and both the homozygous and 1420CT heterozygous genotypes exhibited decreased maternal risk of birth of a child with DS in comparison to the 1420TT genotype [52]. A team of Italian researchers [50] investigated two common *TYMS* polymorphisms in 94 DS bearing and 113 control mothers from the population of Italy. These polymorphisms were rs34743033, which is a 28-bp short tandem repeats in the 5′-untranslated region (5′-UTR) that is linked to gene expression levels [54], andrs34489327, which is a 6-bp deletion (1494 ins/del) polymorphism in the 3′-UTR that causes mRNA instability into the cytoplasm [55, 56]. But the result suggested no independent association of these two polymorphic sites with DS birth, but synergistic effect of the combined *MTHFR* 1298 AC/*TYMS* 28-bp 2R/2R genotype resulted in decreased maternal risk. Regarding *DHFR* gene polymorphism, only known study [51], was conducted including 105 DS bearing and 185 control mothers from Brazilian population for rs70991108 which is the presence of a 19-bp ins/del polymorphism, but no association with maternal risk of a DS birth was detected. But the confirmation of these results has not possible due to lack of replication of study in other populations.

13. Discussion and conclusion

Risk factors associated with Down syndrome birth the enigmatic. Both the genetic and environmental and habitual implications are known to be associated with DS birth. Regarding maternal genotypes that may impose risk of chromosome 21 nondisjunction in oocyte is extremely complicated owing to multifactorial nature of chromosome segregation system. It includes genes that are involved directly in chromosome segregation and also, cell cycle regulators, replication and recombination regulators, and metabolism regulators that maintain the optimum nutrient level affecting the genetic and epigenetic environment. In respect to recombination regulators, only gene that has been investigated in maternal genome is PRDM9. This study [9] is only known analyses on that gene and is needed to be replicated in other populations. Another gene is APOE that exhibited association with DS birth when APOE4 allele is present. Again very limited study has been conducted in this regard. Rest of the genes that have analyses so far in maternal genome for association with DS child are from folate metabolism regulators. Since the initial publication [17] on relation between DS birth risk and folate metabolism regulator polymorphisms in the year1999, several studies on different ethnic populations have been carried and the results are conflicting. But considering the gene X environment concept, it can be justified. The defects in folate metabolism pathways can only be manifested in term of chromosome segregation errors when genetic background interacts with nutritional status of the women. As the genetic background is different for different ethnic populations and as the nutritional level vary according to social architecture of given population, the association study gives different and contradictory results. Moreover, level of folic acid in grand maternal genome is of scientific concern as the oocytes starts growing in the fetal ovary.

In summary, it can be said that genetic architecture of maternal genome is needed to be explored in relation to prevention of DS child birth. Population specific genetic markers are needed to be developed in order to screen the women prior to their conception to test the genetic susceptibility for DS fetal conception. The biggest break through will come with highest level of application of basic research in biomedical field.

Author details

Sujay Ghosh[1]* and Papiya Ghosh[2]

1 Cytogenetics and Genomics Research Unit, Department of Zoology, University of Calcutta, Kolkata, West Bengal, India

2 Department of Zoology, Bijoy Krishna Girls' College, Howrah, West Bengal, India

*Address all correspondence to: sgzoo@caluniv.ac.in; g.sujoy.g@gmail.com

References

[1] Penrose LS. The relative effects of paternal and maternal age in mongolism. Journal of Genetics. 1933;**88**(1):9-14

[2] Oliver TR, Feingold E, Yu K, Cheung V, Tinker S, Yadav-Shah M, et al. New insights into human nondisjunction of chromosome 21 in oocytes. PLoS Genetics. 2008;**4**(3):e1000033. DOI: 10.1371/journal.pgen.1000033

[3] Ghosh S, Feingold E, Dey SK. Etiology of down syndrome: Evidence for consistent association among altered meiotic recombination, nondisjunction, and maternal age across populations. American Journal of Medical Genetics. Part A. 2009;**149A**(7):1415-1420. DOI: 10.1002/ajmg.a.32932

[4] Ghosh S, Feingold E, Chakraborty S, Dey SK. Telomere length is associated with types of chromosome 21 nondisjunction: A new insight into the maternal age effect on down syndrome birth. Human Genetics. 2010;**127**(4):403-409. DOI: 10.1007/s00439-009-0785-8

[5] Albizua I, Rambo-Martin BL, Allen EG, He W, Amin AS, Sherman SL. Association between telomere length and chromosome 21 nondisjunction in the oocyte. Human Genetics. 2015;**134**(11-12):1263-1270. DOI: 10.1007/s00439-015-1603-0

[6] Hayashi K, Yoshida K, Matsui Y. A histone H3 methyltransferase controls epigenetic events required for meiotic prophase. Nature. 2005;**438**:374-378

[7] Myers S, Freeman C, Auton A, Donnelly P, McVean G. A common sequence motif associated with recombination hot spots and genome instability in humans. Nature Genetics. 2008;**40**:1124-1129

[8] Berg IL, Neumann R, Lam KWG, Sarbajna S, Odenthal-Hesse L, et al. PRDM9 variation strongly influences recombination hot-spot activity and meiotic instability in humans. Nature Genetics. 2010;**42**:859-863

[9] Oliver TR, Middlebrooks C, Harden A, Scott N, Johnson B, Jones J, et al. Variation in the zinc finger of PRDM9 is associated with the absence of recombination along nondisjoined chromosomes 21 of maternal origin. Journal of Down Syndrome & Chromosome Abnormalities. 2016;**2**(2):115. DOI: 10.4172/2472-1115.1000115

[10] Avramopoulos D, Mikkelsen M, Vassilopoulos D, Grigoriadou M, Petersen MB. Apolipoprotein E allele distribution in parents of down's syndrome children. Lancet. 1996;**347**(9005):862-865

[11] Ezquerra M, Ballesta F, Queralt R, Aledo R, Gómez D, Guitart M, et al. Apolipoprotein E epsilon 4 alleles and meiotic origin of non-disjunction in down syndrome children and in their corresponding fathers and mothers. Neuroscience Letters. 1998;**248**(1):1-4

[12] Rengifo L, Gaviria D, Serrano H. APOE gene polymorphisms associated with down syndrome in Colombian populations. Biomédica. 2012;**32**(2):224-232. DOI: 10.1590/S0120-41572012000300010

[13] Petersen MB, Karadima G, Samaritaki M, Avramopoulos D, Vassilopoulos D, Mikkelsen M. Association between presenilin-1 polymorphism and maternal meiosis II errors in down syndrome. American Journal of Medical Genetics. 2000;**93**(5):366-372

[14] Bhaumik P, Ghosh P, Ghosh S, Feingold E, Ozbek U, Sarkar B, et al. Combined association of Presenilin-1

and Apolipoprotein E polymorphisms with maternal meiosis II error in down syndrome births. Genetics and Molecular Biology. 2017;**40**(3):577-585. DOI: 10.1590/1678-4685-GMB-2016-0138

[15] Guenther BD, Sheppard CA, Tran P, Rozen R, Matthews RG, Ludwig ML. The structure and properties of methylenetetrahydrofolate reductase from *Escherichia coli* suggest how folate ameliorates human hyperhomocysteinemia. Nature Structural Biology. 1999;**6**:359-365. DOI: 10.1038/7594

[16] Martínez-Frías ML. The biochemical structure and function of methylenetetrahydrofolate reductase provide the rationale to interpret the epidemiological results on the risk for infants with down syndrome. American Journal of Medical Genetics Part A. 2008;**146A**:1477-1482. DOI: 10.1002/ajmg.a.32308

[17] James SJ, Pogribna M, Pogribny IP, Melnyk S, Hine RJ, Gibson JB, et al. Abnormal folate metabolism and mutation in the methylenetetrahydrofolate reductase gene may be maternal risk factors for down syndrome. The American Journal of Clinical Nutrition. 1999;**70**:495-501

[18] Costa-Lima MA, Amorim MR, Orioli IM. Association of methylenetetrahydrofolate reductase gene 677C>T polymorphism and down syndrome. Molecular Biology Reports. 2013;**40**:2115-2125. DOI: 10.1007/s11033-012-2270-z

[19] Wu X, Wang X, Chan Y, Jia S, Luo Y, Tang W. Folate metabolism gene polymorphisms MTHFR C677T and A1298C and risk for down syndrome offspring: A meta-analysis. European Journal of Obstetrics, Gynecology, and Reproductive Biology. 2013;**167**:154-159. DOI: 10.1016/j.ejogrb.2012.11.022

[20] Yang M, Gong T, Lin X, Qi L, Guo Y, Cao Z, et al. Maternal gene polymorphisms involved in folate metabolism and the risk of having a down syndrome offspring: A meta-analysis. Mutagenesis. 2013;**28**:661-671. DOI: 10.1093/mutage/get045

[21] Rai V, Yadav U, Kumar P, Yadav SK, Mishra OP. Maternal methylenetetrahydrofolate reductase C677T polymorphism and down syndrome risk: A meta-analysis from 34 studies. PLoS One. 2014;**9**:e108552. DOI: 10.1371/journal.pone.0108552

[22] Victorino DB, Godoy MF, Goloni-Bertollo EM, Pavarino EC. Meta-analysis of methylenetetrahydrofolate reductase maternal gene in down syndrome: Increased susceptibility in women carriers of the MTHFR 677T allele. Molecular Biology Reports. 2014;**41**:5491-5504. DOI: 10.1007/s11033-014-3424-y

[23] Coppedè F, Grossi E, Migheli F, Migliore L. Polymorphisms in folate-metabolizing genes, chromosome damage, and risk of Down syndrome in Italian women: Identification of key factors using artificial neural networks. BMC Med Genomics. 2010;**3**:42. DOI 10.1186/1755-8794-3-42

[24] Coppedè F. The complex relationship between folate/homocysteine metabolism and risk of down syndrome. Mutation Research. 2019;**682**:54-70. DOI: 10.1016/j.mrrev.2009.06.001

[25] Coppedè F, Colognato R, Bonelli A, Astrea G, Bargagna S, Siciliano G, et al. Polymorphisms in folate and homocysteine metabolizing genes and chromosome damage in mothers of down syndrome children. American Journal of Medical Genetics Part A. 2007;**143A**:2006-2015. DOI: 10.1002/ajmg.a.31886

[26] Grillo LB, Acácio GL, Barini R, Pinto W Jr, Bertuzzo CS. Mutations

in the methylene-tetrahydrofolate reductase gene and down syndrome. Cadernos de Saúde Pública. 2002;**18**:1795-1797. DOI: 10.1590/S0102-311X2002000600035

[27] Acácio GL, Barini R, Bertuzzo CS, Couto EC, Annichino-Bizzacchi M, Júnior WP. Methylenetetrahydrofolate reductase gene polymorphisms and their association with trisomy 21. Prenatal Diagnosis. 2005;**25**:1196-1199. DOI: 10.1002/pd.1296

[28] Scala I, Granese B, Sellitto M, Salomè S, Sammartino A, Pepe A, et al. Analysis of seven maternal polymorphisms of genes involved in homocysteine/folate metabolism and risk of down syndrome offspring. Genetics in Medicine. 2006;**8**:409-416. DOI: 10.1097/01.gim.0000228206.21793.82

[29] Brandalize AP, Bandinelli E, dos Santos PA, Roisenberg I, Schüler-Faccini L. Evaluation of C677T and A1298C polymorphisms of the MTHFR gene as maternal risk factors for down syndrome and congenital heart defects. American Journal of Medical Genetics Part A. 2009;**149A**:2080-2087. DOI: 10.1002/ajmg.a.32989

[30] Zampieri BL, Biselli JM, Goloni-Bertollo EM, Vannucchi H, Carvalho VM, Cordeiro JA, et al. Maternal risk for down syndrome is modulated by genes involved in folate metabolism. Disease Markers. 2012;**32**:73-81. DOI: 10.1155/2012/693864

[31] Hobbs CA, Sherman SL, Yi P, Hopkins SE, Torfs CP, Hine RJ, et al. Polymorphisms in genes involved in folate metabolism as maternal risk factors for down syndrome. American Journal of Human Genetics. 2000;**67**:623-630. DOI: 10.1086/303055

[32] Medica I, Maver A, Goncalo Figueiredo A, Peterlin B. Polymorphisms in genes involved in folate metabolism as maternal risk factors for down syndrome—Meta-analysis. Central European Journal of Medicine. 2009;**4**:395-408. DOI: 10.2478/s11536-009-0055-0

[33] BalduinoVictorino D, de Godoy MF, Goloni-Bertollo EM, Pavarino ÉC. Genetic polymorphisms involved in folate metabolism and maternal risk for down syndrome: A meta-analysis. Disease Markers. 2014;**2014**:517504. DOI: 10.1155/2014/517504

[34] Coppedè F. The genetics of folate metabolism and maternal risk of birth of a child with down syndrome and associated congenital heart defects. Frontiers in Genetics. 2015;**6**:223. DOI: 10.3389/fgene.2015.00223

[35] Wang SS, Qiao FY, Feng L, Lv JJ. Polymorphisms in genes involved in folate metabolism as maternal risk factors for down syndrome in China. Journal of Zhejiang University Science B. 2008;**9**(2):93-99. DOI: 10.1631/jzus.B0710599

[36] Wang SS, Wang C, Qiao FY, Lv JJ, Feng L. Polymorphisms in genes RFC-1/CBS as maternal risk factors for down syndrome in China. Archives of Gynecology and Obstetrics. 2013;**288**:273-277. DOI: 10.1007/s00404-013-2760-9

[37] Bosco P, Guéant-Rodriguez RM, Anello G, Barone C, Namour F, Caraci F, et al. Methionine synthase (MTR) 2756 (A > G) polymorphism, double heterozygosity methionine synthase 2756 AG/methionine synthase reductase (MTRR) 66 AG, and elevated homocysteinemia are three risk factors for having a child with down syndrome. American Journal of Medical Genetics Part A. 2003;**121A**:219-224. DOI: 10.1002/ajmg.a.20234

[38] Coppedè F, Bosco P, Tannorella P, Romano C, Antonucci I, Stuppia L, et al. DNMT3B promoter polymorphisms and maternal risk of birth of a child with down syndrome. Human Reproduction. 2013;**28**:545-550. DOI: 10.1093/humrep/des376

[39] Liao YP, Bao MS, Liu CQ, Liu H, Zhang D. Folate gene polymorphism and the risk of down syndrome pregnancies in young Chinese women. Yi Chuan. 2010;**32**:461-466. DOI: 10.3724/SP.J.1005.2010.00461

[40] Brandalize AP, Bandinelli E, Dos Santos PA, Schüler-Faccini L. Maternal gene polymorphisms involved in folate metabolism as risk factors for down syndrome offspring in Southern Brazil. Disease Markers. 2010;**29**:95-101. DOI: 10.1155/2010/250324

[41] Hou Z, Matherly LH. Biology of the major facilitative folate transporters SLC19A1 and SLC46A1. Current Topics in Membranes. 2014;**73**:175-204. DOI: 10.1016/b978-0-12-800223-0.00004-9

[42] Chango A, Fillon-Emery N, Mircher C, Bléhaut H, Lambert D, Herbeth B, et al. No association between common polymorphisms in genes of folate and homocysteine metabolism and the risk of down's syndrome among French mothers. The British Journal of Nutrition. 2005;**94**:166-169. DOI: 10.1079/BJN20051490

[43] Coppedè F, Marini G, Bargagna S, Stuppia L, Minichilli F, Fontana I, et al. Folate gene polymorphisms and the risk of down syndrome pregnancies in young Italian women. American Journal of Medical Genetics Part A. 2006;**140**:1083-1091. DOI: 10.1002/ajmg.a.31217

[44] Sperandeo MP, de Franchis R, Andria G, Sebastio G. A 68-bp insertion found in a homocystinuric patient is a common variant and is skipped by alternative splicing of the cystathionine beta-synthase mRNA. American Journal of Human Genetics. 1996;**59**:1391-1393

[45] Shao Y, Zhang CG, Cui JH. Association of plasma homocysteine and cystathionine beta-synthase polymorphism with cerebral thrombosis. Di Yi Jun Yi Da Xue Xue Bao. 2005;**25**:351-353

[46] Zampieri BL, Biselli JM, Goloni-Bertollo EM, Pavarino EC. BHMT G742A and MTHFD1 G1958A polymorphisms and down syndrome risk in the Brazilian population. Genetic Testing and Molecular Biomarkers. 2012;**16**:628-631. DOI: 10.1089/gtmb.2011.0257

[47] Izci Ay O, Ay ME, Erdal ME, Cayan F, Tekin S, Soylemez F, et al. Folate metabolism gene polymorphisms and risk for down syndrome offspring in Turkish women. Genetic Testing and Molecular Biomarkers. 2015;**19**:191-197. DOI: 10.1089/gtmb.2014.0262

[48] von Castel-Dunwoody KM, Kauwell GP, Shelnutt KP, Vaughn JD, Griffin ER, Maneval DR, et al. Transcobalamin 776C->G polymorphism negatively affects vitamin B-12 metabolism. The American Journal of Clinical Nutrition. 2005;**81**(6):1436-1441. DOI: 10.1093/ajcn/81.6.1436

[49] Fintelman-Rodrigues N, Corrêa JC, Santos JM, Pimentel MM, Santos-Rebouças CB. Investigation of CBS, MTR, RFC-1 and TC polymorphisms as maternal risk factors for down syndrome. Disease Markers. 2009;**26**:155-161. DOI: 10.1155/2009/504625

[50] Jaiswal SK, Sukla KK, Kumari N, Lakhotia AR, Kumar A, Rai AK. Maternal risk for down syndrome and polymorphisms in the promoter region of the DNMT3B gene: A case-control study. Birth Defects Research Part A: Clinical and Molecular

Teratology. 2015;**103**:299-305. DOI: 10.1002/bdra.23348

[51] Coppedè F, Migheli F, Bargagna S, Siciliano AI, Stuppia L, et al. Association of maternal polymorphisms in folate metabolizing genes with chromosome damage and risk of down syndrome offspring. Neuroscience Letters. 2009;**449**:15-19. DOI: 10.1016/j.neulet.2008.10.074

[52] Mendes CC, Biselli JM, Zampieri BL, Goloni-Bertollo EM, Eberlin MN, Haddad R, et al. 19-base pair deletion polymorphism of the dihydrofolate reductase (DHFR) gene: Maternal risk of down syndrome and folate metabolism. São Paulo Medical Journal. 2010;**128**:215-218. DOI: 10.1590/S1516-31802010000400008

[53] Marucci GH, Zampieri BL, Biselli JM, Valentin S, Bertollo EM, Eberlin MN, et al. Polymorphism C1420T of serine hydroxymethyltransferase gene on maternal risk for down syndrome. Molecular Biology Reports. 2012;**39**:2561-2566. DOI: 10.1007/s11033-011-1008-7

[54] Woeller CF, Anderson DD, Szebenyi DM, Stover PJ. Evidence for small ubiquitin-like modifier-dependent nuclear import of the thymidylate biosynthesis pathway. The Journal of Biological Chemistry. 2007;**282**:17623-17631. DOI: 10.1074/jbc.M702526200

[55] Horie N, Aiba H, Oguro K, Hojo H, Takeishi K. Functional analysis and DNA polymorphism of the tandemly repeated sequences in the 5′-terminal regulatory region of the human gene for thymidylate synthase. Cell Structure and Function. 1995;**20**:191-197. DOI: 10.1247/csf.20.191

[56] Ulrich CM, Bigler J, Bostick R, Fosdick L, Potter JD. Thymidylate synthase promoter polymorphism, interaction with folate intake, and risk of colorectal adenomas. Cancer Research. 2002;**62**:3361-3364

Chapter 5

Current Cytogenetic Abnormalities in Acute Myeloid Leukemia

Mounia Bendari, Nisrine Khoubila, Siham Cherkaoui, Nezha Hda, Meryem Qachouh, Mouna Lamchahab and Asmaa Quessar

Abstract

Cytogenetic abnormalities are frequently reported in the literature describing the presence of chromosomal rearrangements in important cases of acute myeloid leukemia (AML); the rate can reach 50–60% of cases of AML. Cytogenetic abnormalities represent an important prognosis factor, their analysis is crucial for AML; cytogenetic study permits to classify prognostic groups and indicate the treatment strategy and helps to improve the outcome of these patients and to increase their chances of cure. Hundreds of uncommon chromosomal aberrations from AML exist. This chapter summarizes chromosomal abnormalities that are common and classifies AML according to the World Health Organization (WHO) classifications from 2008 to 2016; we will discuss briefly gene mutations detected in normal karyotype (NK) AML by cutting-edge next-generation sequencing technology, like FLT3-ITD, nucleophosmin (NPM1), CCAAT/enhancer-binding protein alpha (CEBPA), and other additional mutations.

Keywords: cytogenetic abnormalities, acute myeloid leukemia, karyotype

1. Introduction

Acute myeloid leukemia (AML) is characterized by clonal expansion of undifferentiated myeloid precursors, resulting in impaired hematopoiesis and bone marrow failure [1].

The discovery of specific chromosomal abnormalities has proved that leukemia is a genetic disease on the cellular level and has also guided the way to mapping and cloning of genes involved in the leukemic process.

The frequency of cytogenetic abnormalities is reported in the literature describing the presence of chromosomal rearrangements in important cases of AML; they are recognized in approximately 56% of de novo AML in adults [2, 3], and the rate can reach 70–80% of the cases of AML in children [4, 5]. At present, cytogenetic aberrations detected at the time of AML diagnosis constitute the most common basis for predicting clinical outcome [6].

Karyotype analysis must be performed as part of the standard diagnostic procedure of AML and have to be reported according to the International System for Nomenclature in Human Cytogenetic (ISCN) 3.

AML appears as a complex and evaluative disease [7, 8]. There are many leukemia genes, most of which are infrequently mutated, and patients typically have more than one driver mutation. The AML evolved over time, with multiple competing clones coexisting at any time [7, 8].

The analysis of cytogenetic abnormalities is indispensable for AML; it represents the most important prognosis factor for patients with AML. In fact, cytogenetic study helps to classify prognosis groups and guide the treatment strategy and permits to improve the outcome of these patients and to increase their chances of cure.

Many uncommon chromosomal aberrations from AML exist. This chapter resumes chromosomal abnormalities that are common in structural and numerical aberrations. Cytogenetic and mutational data are used to divide patients into subgroups defined according to prognostic factors and factors that dictate whether allogeneic hematopoietic stem cell transplantation should be performed during an initial remission.

2. Recurrent cytogenetic abnormalities

2.1 The t(8;21) (q22;q22.1); *RUNX1-RUNX1T1*

The t(8;21) (q22;q22.1); *RUNX1-RUNX1T1* abnormality is considered as a subset with particular clinical and biological specificities. This translocation is defined by fusion between the AML1 gene (RUNX1) on chromosome 21 and the ETO gene (this translocation can be referred to as the RUNX1T1 gene that encodes the CBFA2T1 protein) on chromosome 8. The t(8;21) abnormality is found in approximately 5–10% of all AML cases and 10–22% of AML cases with maturation corresponding to the previous FAB class M2. The t(8;21) generates two fusion genes, AML1-ETO and ETO-AML1, but only the AML1-ETO transcript transcribed from the derivative chromosome 8 is detectable by reverse transcriptase polymerase chain reaction (RT-PCR). Patients with t(8,21) are included in the favorable group; the prognosis after intensive chemotherapy is better for these patients than for the majority of AML patients. The incidence of t(8;21) decreases with age; it is most common in children/younger patients and uncommon in patients above 60 years of age. Approximately 10–20% of children with AML have this translocation [9].

2.2 The inv(16) (p13.1q22) or t(16;16)(p13.1;q22); *CBFB-MYH11*

Approximately 5–7% of acute myeloid leukemia patients have an inv(16) (p13;q22) or t(16;16)(p13;q22). Molecularly, inv(16)/t(16;16) is the result of the juxtaposition of the myosin, heavy chain 11, smooth muscle gene (MYH11) at 16p13 and the core-binding factor, β subunit gene (CBFB) at 16q22; this juxtaposition creates the CBFB-MYH11 fusion gene. The genomic breakpoints can be variable within CBFB and MYH11; this variability explains why in the literature many differently sized CBFB-MYH11 fusion transcript variants have been reported. Type A is the more frequent type of fusion reported; it represents more than 85% of fusions, and 5–10% of each are type D and type E fusions. This cytogenetic group is characterized by its usually association with high complete remission (CR) rates and a relatively favorable outcome [10].

2.3 Acute promyelocytic leukemia with *PML-RARA*

The of reciprocal translocations (15;17) are usually present on acute promyelocytic leukemia (APL); this translocation involves the *PML* gene on 15q24 and *RARA* gene on 17q21 in more than 90% of cases. *PML-RARA* fusion gene results on the derivative chromosome 15.

PML-RARA fusion can also be a result of cases of complex translocations involving 15, 17, and other partner chromosomes or insertions of 15 into 17 and vice versa. Rare variant translocations involving *RARA* and other partner genes have been reported like *PLZF*, *NPM*, *NuMA*, *STAT5b*, *PRKAR1A*, *FIP1L1*, and *BCOR* [11].

2.4 The t(9;11) (p22;q23)

Acute myeloid leukemia with t(9;11) occurs in 3–5% of cases of AML. The translocation t(9;11) (p22;q23) [subsequently referred to as t(9;11)] in acute myeloid leukemia resulting in the MLL-MLLT3-fusion protein represents the most common translocation involving *MLL.* MLL gene at 11q23 (HRX) encodes a DNA-binding protein that positively regulates expression of target genes, including multiple HOX genes, by methylation of histone H3 lys4/chromatin remodeling [12].

2.5 The t(6;9) (p23;q34)

The translocation t(6;9) is a rare recurring cytogenetic aberration and occurs in 0.7–1.8% of cases of AML. This translocation is the result of the formation of a chimeric fusion gene, DEK-NUP214 (previously known as DEK-CAN). It is associated with a poor prognosis; the remission is achieved in less than 50% of cases after chemotherapy [13].

2.6 The inv(3) (q21q26.2) or t(3;3)(q21;q26.2)

The inv(3) (q21q26.2) or t(3;3)(q21;q26.2) occurring at the long arm of chromosome 3 involves the oncogene EVI1 at 3q26.2 (or its longer form MDS1-EVI1) and RPN1 at 3q21, leading to the RPN1-EVI1 fusion transcript. These abnormalities are considered as a separate entity, characterized by an aggressive clinical behavior. RPN1 can amplify EVI1 expression resulting in increased cell proliferation and may impair cell differentiation and be responsible of hematopoietic cell transformation [14].

2.7 The t(1;22) (p13;q13)

Acute megakaryoblastic leukemia (AMKL) with t(1;22) (p13;q13) is an extremely rare subtype of acute myeloid leukemia that is almost always described in infants. The nonrandom association between t(1;22) (p13;q13) and infant AMKL was reported by Baruchel et al. [15]. Just after that, the fusion gene OTT-MAL was identified in patients with t(1;22).

3. WHO classification for myeloid neoplasm regroups

The World Health Organization (WHO) new classification for myeloid neoplasm regroups clinical cytogenetic and molecular criteria, which were associated with the morphological and immunophenotypic characteristics used in the classification recommended by the French-American-British (FAB) cooperative group [16]. The current update of the WHO classification provides few changes to the existing disease categories. The remaining subcategory AML, not otherwise specified (NOS), pure erythroid leukemia, requires more than 80% immature erythroid precursors with more than 30% proerythroblasts. The most important modification concerned a new category "myeloid neoplasms with germ line predisposition" which has been added.

Table 1 summarizes the update of WHO classification of 2016, and **Table 2** gives more details about the new category "myeloid neoplasms with germ line predisposition" [17].

3.1 AML with recurrent genetic abnormalities

The revisit interested in the molecular basis of the LMA with inv(3) (q21.3; q26.2) or t (3; 3) (q21.3; q26.2) has demonstrated that the repositioning of a GATA2 enhancer element which is the cause of overexpression of the MECOM gene (EVI1) and haploinsufficiency of GATA2 [18, 19].

The revisit added another provisional entity; it is about "AML with BCR-ABL1." Treatment with a tyrosine kinase inhibitor for patients with this abnormality is essential. In some cases, distinguishing from blast phase of chronic myeloid leukemia can be difficult; preliminary data suggest that deletion of antigen receptor genes (immunoglobulin heavy chain and T-cell receptor), IKZF1, and/or CDKN2A would be in favor of the diagnosis of AML rather than chronic myeloid leukemia blast phase [20].

When AML is associated with mutated nucleophosmin (NPM1) or biallelic mutations of CCAAT/enhancer-binding protein alpha (CEBPA), it is recognized as full entities. AML associated with biallelic mutations of CEBPA is the only reported as purveyor for the favorable prognosis [21, 22].

Finally, a new provisional entity "AML with mutated RUNX1" (excluding cases with changes associated with myelodysplasia) has been introduced. It has been associated with distinct clinico-pharmacological features and a poor prognosis [23, 24].

3.2 AML with myelodysplasia-related changes

Many criteria were introduced for this category, like the presence of multilineage dysplasia, preexisting myeloid disorder, and/or myelodysplasia-related cytogenetic changes. The deletion 9q was also removed from the list of myelodysplasia-related cytogenetic changes, this modification was done because del9q is usually associated with t(8;21), and it also frequently occurs in AML with NPM1 and biallelic CEBPA mutations [25, 26].

3.3 AML, not otherwise specified

The subgroup with acute erythroid leukemia and erythroid/myeloid type was defined, in the past, by the presence of more than 50% bone marrow erythroid precursors and more than 20% myeloblasts among nonerythroid cells; actually myeloblasts are always counted as percentage of total marrow cells. The remaining subcategory AML, not otherwise specified, pure erythroid leukemia, is defined by the presence of 80% immature erythroid precursors with more than 30% proerythroblasts. On AML NOS, FAB classification does not give any prognosis information if NMP1 and CEBPA documentation are done [27].

3.4 Myeloid neoplasms with germ line predisposition (synonyms: familial myeloid neoplasms; familial myelodysplastic syndromes/acute leukemias)

This new category was recently included; this category needs special investigations from physicians. He must reconstitute the patient and family history.

Myeloid neoplasms with germ line predisposition (see Table 2)	
AML and related neoplasms	**AML and related neoplasms (cont'd)**
AML with recurrent genetic abnormalities	Acute myelomonocytic leukemia
AML with t(8;21)(q22;q22.1); *RUNX1-RUNX1T1*	Acute monoblastic/monocytic leukemia
AML with inv(16)(p13.1q22) or t(16;16)(p13.1;q22); *CBFB-MYH11*	Pure erythroid leukemia[#]
Acute promyelocytic leukemia with *PML-RARA*[*]	Acute megakaryoblastic leukemia
AML with t(9;11)(p21.3;q23.3); *MLLT3-KMT2A*[†]	Acute basophilic leukemia
AML with t(6;9)(p23;q34.1); *DEK-NUP214*	Acute panmyelosis with myelofibrosis
AML with inv(3)(q21.3q26.2) or t(3;3)(q21.3;q26.2); *GATA2,MECOM(EVI1)*	Myeloid sarcoma
AML (megakaryoblastic) with t(1;22)(p13.3;q13.3); *RBM15-MKL1*[‡]	Myeloid proliferations related to Down syndrome
Provisional entity: AML with *BCR-ABL1*	Transient abnormal myelopoiesis
AML with mutated *NPM1*[§]	Myeloid leukemia associated with Down syndrome
AML with biallelic mutations of *CEBPA*[§]	Blastic plasmacytoid dendritic cell neoplasm
Provisional entity: AML with mutated *RUNX1*	**Acute leukemias of ambiguous lineage**
AML with myelodysplasia-related changes[ǀ]	Acute undifferentiated leukemia
Therapy-related myeloid neoplasms[¶]	MPAL with t(9;22)(q34.1;q11.2); *BCR-ABL1*[**]
AML, NOS	MPAL with t(v;11q23.3); *KMT2A* rearranged
AML with minimal differentiation	MPAL, B/myeloid, NOS
AML without maturation	MPAL, T/myeloid, NOS
AML with maturation	

For a diagnosis of AML, a marrow blast count of ≥20% is required, except for AML with the recurrent genetic abnormalities t(15;17), t(8;21), inv(16), or t(16;16).
MPAL, mixed phenotype acute leukemia; NK, natural killer.
[*]*Other recurring translocations involving RARA should be reported accordingly: for example, AML with t(11;17)(q23;q12); ZBTB16-RARA; AML with t(11;17)(q13;q12); NUMA1-RARA; AML with t(5;17)(q35;q12); NPM1-RARA; or AML with STAT5B-RARA (the latter having a normal chromosome 17 on conventional cytogenetic analysis).*
[†]*Other translocations involving KMT2A (MLL) should be reported accordingly: for example, AML with t(6;11)(q27;q23.3); MLLT4-KMT2A; AML with t(11;19)(q23.3;p13.3); KMT2A-MLLT1; AML with t(11;19)(q23.3;p13.1); KMT2A-ELL; and AML with t(10;11)(p12;q23.3); MLLT10-KMT2A.*
[‡]*Rare leukemia most commonly occurring in infants.*
[§]*Diagnosis is made irrespective of the presence or absence of multilineage dysplasia.*
[ǀ]*At least 20% (≥20%) blood or marrow blasts and any of the following: previous history of MDS or MDS/MPN; myelodysplasia-related cytogenetic abnormality (see list below); multilineage dysplasia; and the absence of both prior cytotoxic therapy for unrelated disease and aforementioned recurring genetic abnormalities. Cytogenetic abnormalities sufficient to diagnose AML with myelodysplasia-related changes are complex karyotype (defined as three or more chromosomal abnormalities in the absence of one of the WHO-designated recurring translocations or inversions, that is, t(8;21), inv(16) or t(16;16), t(9;11), t(v;11)(v;q23.3), t(6;9), inv(3) or t(3;3); AML with BCR-ABL1); unbalanced abnormalities: −7 or del(7q); −5 or del(5q); i(17q) or t(17p); −13 or del(13q); del(11q); del(12p) or t(12p); idic(X)(q13); and balanced abnormalities: t(11;16)(q23.3;p13.3); t(3;21)(q26.2;q22.1); t(1;3)(p36.3;q21.2); t(2;11)(p21;q23.3); t(5;12)(q32;p13.2); t(5;7)(q32;q11.2); t(5;17)(q32;p13.2); t(5;10)(q32;q21.2); t(3;5)(q25.3;q35.1).*
[¶]*Cases should be classified with the related genetic abnormality given in the diagnosis.*
[#]*The former subgroup of acute erythroid leukemia and erythroid/myeloid type (≥50% bone marrow erythroid precursors and ≥ 20% myeloblasts among nonerythroid cells) was removed; myeloblasts are now always counted as percentage of total marrow cells. The remaining subcategory AML, NOS, pure erythroid leukemia, requires the presence of >80% immature erythroid precursors with ≥30% proerythroblasts.*
[**]*BCR-ABL1+ leukemia may present as MPAL; treatment should include a tyrosine kinase inhibitor.*

Table 1.
Myeloid neoplasms with germ line predisposition, AML and related precursor neoplasms, and acute leukemias of ambiguous lineage (WHO 2016).

WHO classification
Classification*
Myeloid neoplasms with germ line predisposition without a preexisting disorder or organ dysfunction
AML with germ line *CEBPA* mutation
Myeloid neoplasms with germ line *DDX41* mutation†
Myeloid neoplasms with germ line predisposition and preexisting platelet disorders
Myeloid neoplasms with germ line *RUNX1* mutation†
Myeloid neoplasms with germ line *ANKRD26* mutation†
Myeloid neoplasms with germ line *ETV6* mutation†
Myeloid neoplasms with germ line predisposition and other organ dysfunction
Myeloid neoplasms with germ line *GATA2* mutation
Myeloid neoplasms associated with bone marrow failure syndromes
Juvenile myelomonocytic leukemia associated with neurofibromatosis, Noonan syndrome, or Noonan syndrome-like disorders
Myeloid neoplasms associated with Noonan syndrome
Myeloid neoplasms associated with Down syndrome†
Guide for molecular genetic diagnostics‡
Myelodysplastic predisposition/acute leukemia predisposition syndromes
CEBPA, *DDX41*, *RUNX1*, *ANKRD26*, *ETV6*, *GATA2*, *SRP72*, 14q32.2 genomic duplication (*ATG2B*/*GSKIP*)
Cancer predisposition syndromes§
Li-Fraumeni syndrome (*TP53*)
Germ line *BRCA1*/*BRCA2* mutations
Bone marrow failure syndromes
Dyskeratosis congenita (*TERC*, *TERT*)
Fanconi anemia

**Recognition of familial myeloid neoplasms requires that physicians take a thorough patient and family history to assess for typical signs and symptoms of known syndromes, including data on malignancies and previous bleeding episodes.*
†Lymphoid neoplasms are also reported.
‡Molecular genetic diagnostics are guided by a detailed patient and family history; diagnostics should be performed in close collaboration with a genetic counselor; patients with a suspected heritable myeloid neoplasm, who test negative for known predisposition genes, should ideally be entered on a research study to facilitate new syndrome discovery.
§Mutations in genes associated with cancer predisposition genes such as TP53 and BRCA1/2 appear to be frequent in therapy-related myeloid neoplasms.

Table 2.
WHO classification of myeloid neoplasms with germ line predisposition and guide for molecular genetic diagnostics.

Affected patients, including their families, should benefit from genetic counseling with a counselor familiar with these disorders.

4. European leukemia net 2017 recommendations

The WHO 2008 and 2016 classifications incorporated modifications that allowed for a greater number of patients to be classified into the category of AML [28]. However, in 2010, an international expert panel, on behalf of the European

Leukemia Net (ELN), established recommendations for diagnosis and management of acute myeloid leukemia. These recommendations have been widely used in practice, within clinical trials, and by regulatory agencies. Recently, a big progress has been made in understanding disease pathogenesis and in the development of diagnostic assays and novel therapies. The ELN recommendations were updated, and new recommendations were published.

The goal of ELN is to subdivide genetic categories on prognostic groups to make easier correlations between genetic abnormalities and clinical characteristics and outcomes.

Although a subsequent study elicited a longer overall survival (OS) in the intermediate I group than in the intermediate II group, both groups were prognostically indistinguishable in the more aged patients, who represent the majority of AML cases [25].

The new recommendation of ELN identifies three groups (favorable, intermediate, adverse) with some changes. It was proved that in AML with NPM1 or biallelic CEBPA mutations, the presence of coexisting chromosomal abnormalities does not appear to modify the prognostic [29].

The latest published research has confirmed that the relapse rate and outcomes associated with FLT3-ITD are related to the ITD allele ratio. Studies showed that patients with NPM1 and FLT3-ITD mutation with a low allelic ratio (<0.5) (FLT3-ITDlow) have the same response rate as patients with NPM1 mutation but no FLT3-ITD; they are classified in the favorable group.

The latest findings from recent research suggest that the presence of the FLT3 mutation alone is not sufficient to classify patients into unfavorable prognostic groups and that patients with a NPM1 and FLT3-ITD mutation with a low allelic ratio (<0.5) (FLT3-ITDlow) have the same result as patients with a NPM1 mutation without FLT3-ITD; they are included in a favorable group [30, 31].

Patients with a high ratio are classified in the unfavorable group when they have wild-type NPM1 and FLT3-ITD with a high (>0.5) allelic ratio (FLT3-ITD^{high}); those patients have a poor outcome, but recently the use of FLT3 inhibitors can improve prognosis [32].

Other abnormalities were introduced to adverse-risk group like RUNX1, ASXL1, and TP53 mutations and monosomal karyotype [33, 34].

5. Medical Research Council (MRC) cytogenetic classification

In the past Medical Research Council (MRC) cytogenetic classification was developed, by analyzing a cohort of 1612 children and younger adults (55 years) treated in the MRC AML10 trial; this work was realized more than a decade ago and distinguishes three cytogenetic risk groups [35]. The first group includes patients with t(15;17), t(8;21), and inv(16), irrespective of the presence of additional cytogenetic changes; these categories were assigned to the "favorable-risk" group. The 2sd group concerns patients who have none of these aberrations and who have abn(3q), del (5q), 5/7, or complex karyotype (five or more unbound cytogenetic abnormalities). This group was considered as an "adverse risk." Other patients, those with normal karyotype (NK) and other structural or numerical abnormalities, were in the "intermediate-risk" group. In the original MRC study, patients having infrequent or rare abnormalities were not considered individually and were assigned to the intermediate-risk group [36].

Advances in molecular biology have provided important insights into molecular abnormalities that previously were poorly understood.

Significant advances in technology, including chromosome banding, with fluorescence/chromosome in situ hybridization, or other analyses like array comparative network genomic hybridization, genome breakpoints cloning and Sanger sequencing of candidate genes and profiling of single nucleotide polymorphism, and even whole-genome sequencing (WGS), whole-exome sequencing (WES), and RNA sequencing have all contributed to incremental improvements in understanding the genetic basis of the AML.

The whole-genome sequencing for AML confirmed that it is a complex and instable disease. There are many leukemia genes, most of which are infrequently mutated, and patients typically have many driver mutations. The evolution is characterized by emergence of many competing clones which can coexist at any time.

Figure 1 illustrates different genes and clones coexisting in the same patient [17].

The Cancer Genome Atlas (TCGA) consortium analyzed 200 AML patients by whole-genome or whole-exome sequencing and identified 23 genes as "significantly mutated" at a higher-than-expected frequency [37].

Recently research confirmed that normal karyotype AML is a very heterogeneous group; many gene mutations were detected in normal karyotype AML by cutting-edge next-generation sequencing NGS technology, like FLT3-ITD, NPM1, CEBPA, and other additional mutations.

DNMT3A and RUNX1 mutations represent the most important predictors of shorter overall survival in AML patients aged less than 60 years and particularly in those with intermediate-risk cytogenetic. NPM1 mutations in the absence of FLT3-ITD, mutated TP53, and biallelic CEBPA mutations were identified as important molecular prognosticators of OS irrespective of patient age. Researching these gene mutations is important. It can be helpful on diagnosis and it can be a molecular marker of prognosis, predictive for response of treatment, and used also for disease monitoring.

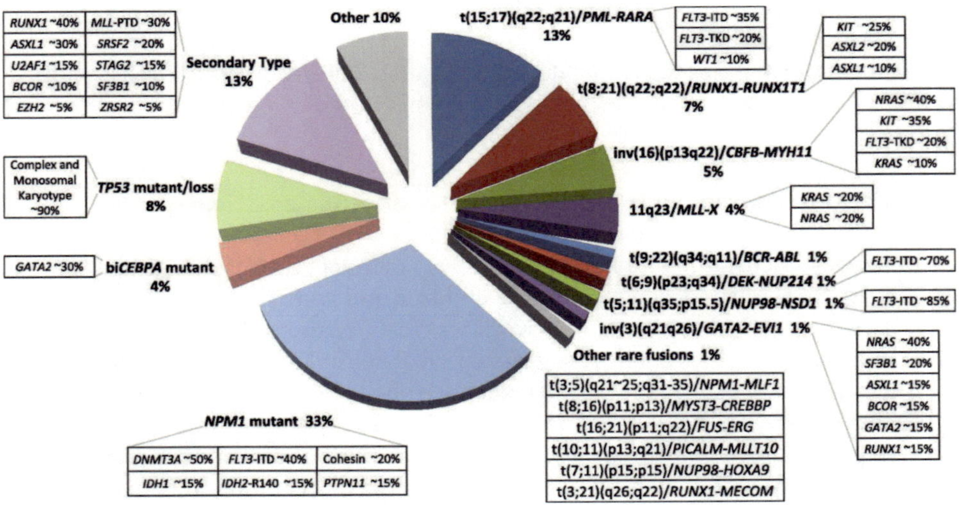

Figure 1.

Molecular classes of AML and concurrent gene mutations in adult patients up to the age of ~65 years. For each AML class denoted in the pie chart, frequent co-occurring mutations are shown in the respective boxes. Data on the frequency of genetic lesions are compiled from the databases of the British Medical Research Council (MRC) and the German-Austrian AML study group (AMLSG) and from selected studies. It indicates cohesin genes including RAD21 (10%), SMC1A (5%), and SMC3 (5%); inv(16)(p13.1q22) or t(16;16)(p13.1;q22); CBFB-MYH11; and inv(3)(q21.3q26.2) or t(3;3)(q21.3;q26.2); GATA2,MECOM(EVI1), and TP53 mutations are found in 45% and complex karyotypes in 70% of this class.

It has been proven in previous studies that patients with cytogenetically normal AML or intermediate-risk abnormalities have more additional gene mutations than patients with favorable or unfavorable abnormal cytogenetic and especially those with balanced translocations [38].

Elderly patients have more driver gene mutations than younger patients. Older patients are characterized by having more alterations in specific genes including TET2, RUNX1, ASXL1, and SRSF2. All this genes have recently been implicated in age-related clonal hematopoiesis. These data contribute to highlight our understanding of differences in AML biology between younger and older patients [39].

5.1 Mutations in the fms-related tyrosine kinase 3 gene (*FLT3*)

Mutations in the fms-related tyrosine kinase 3 gene (*FLT3*) are present in 30% of patients having AML [40]. In approximately three quarters of these patients, the mutation found concerns *FLT3* internal tandem duplication mutation (ITD subtype). This mutation is the result of the duplication between 3 and more than 100 amino acids located in the juxtamembrane region. Studies confirmed that patients with AML having ITD mutations had a poor outcome with high risk to relapse. The rate of response is related to the ratio of mutant. In fact, the prognosis is poorer when there is a high ratio of mutant to wild-type *FLT3* alleles. This permits the development of specific treatment of such FLT3 inhibitors.

In fact, recent studies showed that the use of several specific tyrosine kinase inhibitors improves outcome and clinical trials that are underway [41, 42]. The inclusion of such inhibitors in therapeutic strategy with alloHCT might further improve future outcome of patients with FLT3-ITD AML [43].

5.2 Nucleophosmin protein mutation

NPM1 mutation is detected approximately in 30% of cases of AML with normal karyotype NPM; it is an aberrant cytoplasmic localization of the nucleoplasmin protein. Nuclephosmin protein mutation also named as B23 or numatrin, is a nucleocytoplasmic shuttling protein that constantly exchanges between the nucleus and cytoplasm [44].

5.3 CCAAT/enhancer-binding protein alpha mutations

CCAAT/enhancer-binding protein alpha mutations in AML are associated with favorable prognosis and are divided into N- and C-terminal mutations (double-mutated). CEBPA mutation occurs in 5–10% of cases of acute myeloid leukemia. Recent studies have shown that CEBPA-double-mutated (CEBPA-dm) cases, rather than single mutants, are associated with a common gene expression signature and a relatively favorable outcome. Based on these features, CEBPA-dm AML has been recognized as a separate entity in the revised World Health Organization 2016 classification [45].

5.4 Recurrent mutations in isocitrate dehydrogenase 1/2 (IDH1/IDH2)

Recurrent mutations in isocitrate dehydrogenase 1/2 (IDH1/IDH2) occur in ~12% of patients with acute myeloid leukemia with normal karyotype. Mutated IDH2 proteins neomorphically synthesize 2-hydroxyglutarate resulting in DNA and histone hypermethylation, which leads to blocked cellular differentiation. The incidence of this gene mutation increases with age [46]. Enasidenib (AG-221/CC-90007) and ivosidenib (AG-120) are first-in-class, oral, selective, small-molecule inhibitors of IDH2- and IDH1-mutant enzymes, respectively.

5.5 DNMT3A mutation

DNA methyltransferase (DNMT) 3A catalyzes the addition of methyl groups to the cytosine residue of CpG dinucleotides in DNA; the role of DNMT3A is to encode the DNMT. DNMT3A is constituted by three main structure domains: an ATRX, DNMT3, and DNMT3L-type zinc finger domain, a proline-tryptophan-tryptophan-proline domain, and the methyltransferase (MTase) domain.

The proline-tryptophan-tryptophan-proline domain targets the enzyme to nucleic acid, whereas the zinc finger domain is responsible of mediating protein-protein and interacting with the transcription factors Myc and RP58, the hetero-chromatin protein HP1, histone deacetylases, and the histone methyltransferase Suv39h1 [47].

DNMT3A mutation confers a specific clinical and biological feature, it is associated with poor prognostic, and it represents an unfavorable risk factor in AML patients independent of others risk factors like age, WBC counts, karyotype, and other genetic markers.

6. Conclusion

The update of WHO classification and ELN recommendations is useful for physicians; it can help to better subdivide risk groups and propose adequate treatment for each group [28]. On the other hand, an increasing understanding of molecular aberrations that triggers the development of AML and growing use of next-generation sequencing are advancing the development of investigational drugs against potential driver mutations in AML.

Conflict of interest

The authors declare no conflict of interest.

Author details

Mounia Bendari[1*], Nisrine Khoubila[2], Siham Cherkaoui[2], Nezha Hda[2], Meryem Qachouh[2], Mouna Lamchahab[2] and Asmaa Quessar[2]

1 Mohammed VI University of Health Sciences (UM6SS), Casablanca, Morocco

2 Hematology and Pediatric Oncology Department, Ibn Rochd University Hospital, Casablanca, Morocco

*Address all correspondence to: bendarimounia@gmail.com

References

[1] Creutzig U, van den Heuvel-Eibrink MM, Gibson B, Dworzak MN, Adachi S, de Bont E, et al. Diagnosis and management of acute myeloid leukemia in children and adolescents: Recommendations from an international expert panel. Blood. 2012;**120**:3187-3205

[2] Rooij JD, Zwaan CM, van den Heuvel-Eibrink M. Pediatric AM: From biology to clinical management. Journal of Clinical Medicine. 2015;**4**:127-149

[3] McGowan-Jordan J, Simons A, Scmid M. International Standing Committee on Human Cytogenomic Nomenclature. Karger, Basel, Switzerland: ISCN: An International System for Human Cytogenomic Nomenclature; 2016

[4] Vardiman JW, Thiele J, Arber DA, Brunning RD, Borowitz MJ, Porwit A, et al. The 2008 revision of the World Health Organization (WHO) classification of myeloid neoplasms and acute leukemia: Rationale and important changes. Blood. 2009;**114**(5):937-951

[5] Cheng Y, Wang Y, Wang H, Chen Z, Lou J, Wang H, et al. Cytogenetic Profile of de Novo Acute Myeloid Leukemia: A Study Based on 1432 Patients in a Single Institution of China Leukemia. Vol. 23.2009. pp. 1801-1806

[6] Dohner H, Elihu HE, Amadori S, Appelbaum FR, Buchner T, Burnett AK, et al. Diagnosis and management of acute myeloid leukemia In adults: Recommendations from an international expert panel, on behalf of the European Leukemian. Blood. 2010;**114**:453-474

[7] Grimwade D, Hills RK, Moorman AV, Walker H, Chatters S, Goldstone AH, et al. Refinement of cytogenetic classification in acute myeloid leukemia: Determination of prognostic significance of rare recurring chromosomal abnormalities among 5876 younger adult patients treated In the United Kingdom Medical Research Council trials. Blood. 2010;**116**(3):354-365

[8] Grimwade D, Walker H, Oliver F, et al. On behalf of the Medical Research Council adult and children's leukaemia working parties. The importance of diagnostic Cytogenetics on outcome in AML: Analysis of 1612 patients entered into the MRC AML10 trial. Blood. 1998;**92**(7):2322-2333

[9] Reikvam HK, Hatfield KJ, Kittang AO, Hovland R, Bruserud O. Acute myeloid leukemia with the t(8;21) translocation: Clinical consequences and biological implications Hindawi publishing corporation. Journal of Biomedicine and Biotechnology. **2011**:104631. DOI: 10.1155/2011/104631

[10] Schwind S, Edwards CG, Nicolet D, et al. Inv(16), T(16;16) acute myeloid leukemia with non–type a CBFB-MYH11 fusions associate with distinct clinical and genetic features and lack KIT mutations. Blood. 2013;**121**:385-391

[11] Campbell LJ, Oei P, Brookwell R, Shortt J, Eaddy N, Ng A, et al. FISH detection of PML-RARA fusion in ins(15;17) acute promyelocytic leukaemia depends on probe size Hindawi publishing corporation. BioMed Research International;**2013**:164501

[12] Kühn MW, Bullinger L, Gröschel S, Krönke J, Edelmann J, Rücker FG, et al. Genome-wide genotyping of acute myeloid leukemia with translocation t(9;11)(p22;q23) reveals novel recurrent genomic alterations. Haematologica. 2014;**99**(8):e133-e135

[13] Moraleda PP, Alonzo TA, Gerbing RA, Raimond ISC, et al. Acute myeloid leukemia with t(6;9)(p23;q34) is associated poor outcome in childhood AML regardless of FLT3/ITD status, a report from Children's oncology group. Blood. 2012;**120**:2541

[14] Raya JM et al. Acute myeloid leukemia with Inv(3)(q21;q26.2) or T(3;3)(q21;q26.2). Hematology. 2015;**20**(8):435

[15] Baruchel A, Daniel MT, Schaison G, Berger R. Nonrandom t(1;22) (P12-P13;Q13) in acute megakaryocytic malignant proliferation. Cancer Genetics and Cytogenetics. 1991;**54**:239-243

[16] Grimwade D, Hills RK, Moorman AV, Walker H, Chatters S, et al. Determination of prognostic significance of rare recurring chromosomal abnormalities among 5876 younger adult patients treated in the United Kingdom Medical Research Council trials. Blood. 2010;**116**(3)

[17] Döhner H, Estey E, Grimwade D, Amadori S, Appelbaum FR, Büchner T, et al. Diagnosis and management of AML in adults: 2017 ELN recommendations from an international expert panel. Blood. 2017;**129**(4)

[18] The Cancer Genome Atlas Research Network. Genomic and epigenomic land- scapes of adult de novo acute myeloid leukemia. The New England Journal of Medicine. 2013;**368**:2059-2074

[19] Shlush LI, Zandi S, Mitchell A, et al. Identification of pre-leukaemic haematopoietic stem cells in acute leukaemia. Nature. 2014;**506**:328-333

[20] Papaemmanuil E,Gerstung M, Bullinger L, Gaidzik VI, Paschka P, Roberts ND, et al. Genomic classification and prognosis in acute myeloid leukemia. The New England Journal of Medicine. 2016;**374**(23)

[21] Groschel S, Sanders MA, Hoogenboezem R, et al. A single oncogenic enhancer rearrangement causes concomitant EVI1 and GATA2 deregulation in leukemia. Cell. 2014;**157**(2):369-381

[22] Yamazaki H, Suzuki M, Otsuki A, et al. A remote GATA2 hematopoietic enhancer drives leukemogenesis in inv(3)(q21;q26) by activating EVI1 expression. Cancer Cell. 2014;**25**(4):415-427

[23] Nacheva EP, Grace CD, Brazma D, et al. Does BCR/ABL1 positive acute myeloid leukaemia exist? British Journal of Haematology. 2013;**161**(4):541-550

[24] Wouters BJ, Löwenberg B, Erpelinck-Verschueren CA, van Putten WL, Valk PJ, Delwel R. Double CEBPA mutations, but not single CEBPA mutations, define a subgroup of acute myeloid leukemia with a distinctive gene expression profile that is uniquely associated with a favorable outcome. Blood. 2009;**113**(13):3088-3091

[25] Schlenk RF, Taskesen E, van Norden Y, et al. The value of allogeneic and autologous hematopoietic stem cell transplantation in prognostically favorable acute myeloid leukemia with double mutant CEBPA. Blood. 2013;**122**(9):1576-1582

[26] Tang JL, Hou HA, Chen CY, et al. AML1/RUNX1 mutations in 470 adult patients with De novo acute myeloid leukemia: Prognostic implication and interaction with other gene alterations. Blood. 2009;**114**(26):5352-5361

[27] Haferlach T, Stengel A, Eckstein S, et al. The new provisional WHO entity 'RUNX1 mutated AML' shows specific genetics but no prognostic influence of dysplasia. Leukemia. 2016;**30**(10):2109-2112

[28] Peterson L, Bloomfield CD, Döhner H, Niemeyer C, Godley L. Myeloid neoplasms with germline predisposition. In: Swerdlow S, Campo E, Harris NL, et al., editors. World Health Organization Classification of Tumours of Haematopoietic and Lymphoid Tissues. 4th ed. Lyon, France: World Health Organization;

[29] Haferlach C, Mecucci C, Schnittger S, et al. AML with mutated NPM1 carrying a Normal or aberrant karyotype show overlapping biologic, pathologic, immunophenotypic, and prognostic features. Blood. 2009;**114**(14):3024-3032

[30] Walter RB, Othus M, Burnett AK, et al. Significance of FAB subclassification of "acute myeloid leukemia, NOS" in the 2008 WHO classification: Analysis of 5848 newly diagnosed patients. Blood. 2013;**121**(13):2424-2431

[31] Mrozek K, Marcucci G, Nicolet D, et al. Prognostic significance of the European leukemianet standardized system for reporting cytogenetic and molecular alterations in adults with acute myeloid leukemia. Journal of Clinical Oncology. 2012;**30**(36):4515-4523

[32] Micol JB, Boissel N, Renneville A, et al. The role of cytogenetic abnormalities in acute myeloid leukemia with NPM1 mutations and no FLT3 internal tandem duplication. Blood. 2009;**114**(20):4601-4602

[33] Gale RE, Green C, Allen C, et al. Medical research council adult leukaemia working party. The impact of FLT3 internal tandem duplication mutant level, number, size, and interaction with NPM1 mutations in a large cohort of young adult patients with acute myeloid leukemia. Blood. 2008;**111**(5):2776-2784

[34] Linch DC, Hills RK, Burnett AK, Khwaja A, Gale RE. Impact of FLT3(ITD) mutant allele level on relapse risk In intermediate-risk acute myeloid leukemia. Blood. 2014;**124**(2):273-276

[35] Breems DA, Van Putten WLJ, De Greef GE, et al. Monosomal karyotype in acute myeloid leukemia: A better indicator of poor prognosis than a complex karyotype. Journal of Clinical Oncology. 2008;**26**(29):4791-4797

[36] Pasquini MC, Zhang MJ, Medeiros BC, et al. Hematopoietic cell transplantation outcomes in monosomal karyotype myeloid malignancies. Biology of Blood and Marrow Transplantation. 2016;**22**(2):248-257

[37] Cortes JE, Kantarjian H, Foran JM, et al. Phase I study of quizartinib administered daily to patients with relapsed or refractory acute myeloid leukemia irrespective of FMS-like tyrosine kinase 3-internal tandem duplication status. Journal of Clinical Oncology. 2013;**31**:3681-3687

[38] Galanis A, Ma H, Rajkhowa T, et al. Crenolanib is a potent inhibitor of FLT3 with activity against resistance-conferring point mutants. Blood. 2014;**123**:94-100

[39] Metzelder SK, Schroeder T, Finck A, et al. High activity of Sorafenib in FLT3-ITD-positive acute myeloid leukemia synergizes with allo-immune effects to induce sustained responses. Leukemia. 2012;**26**:2353-2359

[40] Cancer Genome Atlas Research Network. Genomic and epigenomic landscapes of adult de novo acute myeloid leukemia. The New England Journal of Medicine. 2013;**368**(22):2059-2074

[41] Kihara R, Nagata Y, Kiyoi H, et al. Comprehensive analysis of genetic alterations and their prognostic impacts In adult acute myeloid

leukemia patients. Leukemia. 2014;**28**(8):1586-1595

[42] Metzeler KH, Herold T, Rothenberg-Thurley M, Amler S. On behalf of the AMLCG study group spectrum and prognostic relevance of driver gene mutations in acute myeloid leukemia. Blood. 2016;**128**(5)

[43] Kindler T, Lipka DB, Fischer T. FLT3 as a therapeutic target in AML: Still Chal-Lenging after all these years. Blood. 2010;**116**:5089-5102

[44] Borer RA, Lehner CF, Eppenberger HM, Nigg EA. Major nucleolar proteins shuttle between nucleus and cytoplasm. Cell. 1989;**56**:379-390

[45] Mannelli F, Ponziani V, Bencini S, Bonetti MI, et al. *Cebpa*–double-mutated acute myeloid leukemia displays a unique phenotypic profile: A reliable screening method and insight into biological features. Haematologica. 2017;**102**:529-540. DOI: 10.3324/haematol.2016.151910

[46] Brenner C, Fuks F. DNA methyltransferases: Facts, clues, mysteries. Current Topics in Microbiology and Immunology. 2006;**301**:45-66

[47] Chen T, Li E. Establishment and maintenance of DNA methylation patterns in mammals. Current Topics in Microbiology and Immunology. 2006;**301**:179-201

Chapter 6

First-Tier Array CGH in Clinically Variable Entity Diagnosis: 22q13.3 Deletion Syndrome

Magdalena Budisteanu, Andreea Tutulan-Cunita, Ina Ofelia Focsa, Sorina Mihaela Papuc and Aurora Arghir

Abstract

Phelan-McDermid (PMS) or 22q13 deletion syndrome (OMIM 606232) is a rare genetic disorder with highly variable clinical presentation. The phenotype includes generalized neonatal hypotonia, developmental delay with intellectual disability and delayed speech, mild dysmorphic features, and autistic behavior. The genetic defects of PMS consist of 22q13.3 deletions or chromosomal structural rearrangements involving *SHANK3* gene; the loss of function mutations of *SHANK3* gene was reported in a minority of cases. The 22q13.3 deletions vary in size, from 0.2 to over 9 Mb, and, although larger deletions are generally associated with more severe phenotypes, the genotype-phenotype correlations are not clear-cut for all patients. *SHANK3* is considered the main candidate gene for the neurologic features of PMS. PMS is a rare disorder, often underdiagnosed. There are no established clinical diagnostic criteria for PMS. The genetic tests typically used are chromosomal microarray and multiplex ligation-dependent probe amplification (MLPA) or fluorescent in situ hybridization (FISH) for copy number analysis of *SHANK3* gene; next-generation sequencing (NGS) or Sanger sequencing is used for pathogenic mutation screening of *SHANK3*. In this chapter, we report three cases with PMS and summarize the clinical and genetic diagnostic approaches of this condition, highlighting the role of chromosomal microarray technology in the identification of rare, but significantly impacting patient's life, DNA copy number abnormalities.

Keywords: chromosomal microarray, deletions, intellectual disability, speech delay, autistic features

1. Introduction

Phelan-McDermid or 22q13 deletion syndrome (OMIM 606232, PMS) is a genetic disorder characterized by a wide phenotypic spectrum that includes neonatal hypotonia, global developmental delay with cognitive deficits, absent to severely delayed speech (usually, more advanced perceptive language than expressive language), dysmorphic features (dolichocephaly, large or malformed ears, full brows, full cheeks, bulbous nose, pointed chin), behavioral abnormalities with autistic features (poor eye contact, stereotypic movements, impaired social interactions, aggressive behavior), and various neurological problems (reduced perception of pain, seizures, abnormal patterns of movements, habitual chewing or mouthing, inability to regulate sweating) [1–3]. Patients with PMS are highly unlikely to ever function independently. Less often, congenital kidney anomalies [3], arachnoid cysts [1], and higher frequency of other pathological conditions (gastrointestinal disease, upper respiratory tract infections, ventriculomegaly, dysmyelination, morphological changes of the corpus callosum [4]) are described. No life-threatening malformations are associated with this disorder; however, as the number of patients reaching older ages is small, there may be yet a not identified potential for developing life-threatening conditions. Its incidence is not known, but the PMS Foundation estimates approximately 1949 patients worldwide, as of September 2018 on http://www.22q13.org; the prevalence of subjects with PMS in patients with neurodevelopmental delay was estimated at 0.27% [5]; it is present with equal frequency in both sexes.

The genetic anomalies associated with PMS involve 22q13.3 region, leading to *SHANK3* gene haploinsufficiency, in the vast majority of cases. Simple deletions were described in ~79% of patients; deletions generated by unbalanced translocations, ring chromosomes, or complex chromosomal rearrangements were reported in ~18% of patients. In addition, mutations involving *SHANK3* gene were detected in a minority of patients (~3%) with PMS phenotype [6].

Chromosome 22q13.3 deletions range from 0.2 to over 9 Mb [5, 7]. A critical region for PMS was refined in 2002 by Anderlid et al. [8], to 100 kb containing *SHANK3*, *ACR*, and *RABL2B*, with *SHANK3* being the candidate gene for the clinical features of PMS. In 2001, Bonaglia et al. [9] reported a patient with a phenotype consistent with PMS, bearing a translocation t(12;22) which disrupted *SHANK3* gene only. Subsequent studies, reporting small chromosomal deletions and mutations, brought further evidence supporting the role of *SHANK3* gene in PMS neuropsychiatric phenotype [10, 11]. Both contiguous gene deletion at 22q13.3, including SHANK3, and pathogenic variants of *SHANK3* were reported in PMS. Rarely, interstitial deletions with intact *SHANK3* and PMS-like phenotypes have been described, indicating that haploinsufficiency of other genes or a positional effect influencing *SHANK3* expression may cause the same phenotype in some patients [12–14].

SHANK3 encodes for a scaffold protein that connects ion channels and receptors in the postsynaptic density of glutamatergic synaptic membrane to the cytoskeleton, thus participating in a signal transduction pathway highly relevant to various forms of autism spectrum disorder (ASD) [1, 4, 15, 16]. Neurons differentiated from induced pluripotent stem cells from patients with PMS have reduced *SHANK3* expression and major defects in excitatory, but not inhibitory synaptic transmission [17]. Yi et al. [18] demonstrated, in 2016, that *SHANK3* haploinsufficiency decreases I_h channel function, leading to altered synaptic function.

The deletions in PMS patients span a large genomic region and encompass numerous protein coding genes; many of these genes are highly expressed in the brain [19]. Genotype-phenotype correlations connected larger deletion sizes with the severity of the developmental profile, hypotonia, increased number of medical comorbidities, dysmorphic features, and absence of an ASD diagnosis [12]; on the contrary, other studies suggested more severe autistic phenotype in patients with larger deletions, or even no association at all [4]. Additionally, it has been hypothesized that the increase in the deletion size may attenuate the effects of *SHANK3* deficiency, i.e., autistic features, due to additional genes concomitant deletions; also, the severe developmental and language impairments observed in patients with larger deletions make the evaluation of autistic features more difficult [12].

The genetic anomalies in PMS are de novo (80% of cases) or inherited from parents with balanced translocations, inversions, or mosaics (20% of cases); Sarasua et al. [12] reported a 75% inheritance of the abnormal chromosome from the father, but no association with parental age at conception. PMS has been described both in mosaic and non-mosaic forms.

PMS is a rare disorder, with a broad phenotypic spectrum, that often goes underdiagnosed. As there are no specific clinical features suggestive for PMS, the diagnosis is genetic. Chromosomal microarray is the method most commonly used, as a first-tier approach; various techniques can be used for confirmation of copy number imbalance (fluorescent in situ hybridization (FISH), multiplex ligation-dependent probe amplification (MLPA), or qPCR. We report three cases with PMS and summarize the clinical and genetic diagnostic approaches of this condition, highlighting the role of array-based comparative genomic hybridization (array CGH) technology in identification of rare, but significantly impacting patient's life, DNA copy number abnormalities.

2. Materials and methods

Our patients have been referred to clinical and genetic evaluation for developmental delay and behavior problems. The patients have been clinically evaluated by a multidisciplinary team including child psychiatry and child neurology specialists, as well as a psychologist. Array-based comparative genomic hybridization (array CGH) using two oligonucleotide platforms (180 and 60 K) was performed on genomic DNA (gDNA) isolated from peripheral blood, as recommended by manufacturer (Agilent Technologies, Agilent Oligonucleotide Array-Based CGH for Genomic DNA Analysis Enzymatic Labeling for Blood, Cells, or Tissues Protocol, Version 7.3, March 2014). FISH using bacterial artificial chromosome (BAC) probes RP11-316I10 (22q11.21), CTA799F10, and cosmide n85a3 (22q13.33) was carried out according to standard protocol, in probands and parents.

All three patients were born to healthy, non-consanguineous parents, following uncomplicated pregnancies and with no perinatal events. Patients 1 and 2 are siblings; patient 3 is the second child, having a healthy sibling. **Table 1** summarizes the clinical characteristics of our patients.

The first patient, a 4-year-old boy, with a height of 91 cm (Pc 5), weight of 16 kg (Pc 25), and occipitofrontal circumference (OCP) of 49 cm (Pc 25), presented delayed psychomotor development (walked alone at 18 months, says no syllables); minor dysmorphic features: hypoplastic helix, bilateral epicanthus, long eyelashes, and thin upper lip; bilateral 2nd–3rd toes partial cutaneous syndactyly; and sacral dermal sinus. Neurological evaluation revealed gross and fine motor inabilities and absent speech. Psychiatric and psychologic evaluation showed severe intellectual disability, autistic features (absent psychical and visual contact, stereotypic play, no social interactions), and hyperkinesia with aggressive behavior. He had a history of repeated respiratory infections. Electroencephalography (EEG) and abdominal ultrasound investigations were normal. Brain MRI revealed minimal dysmyelination and corpus callosum hypotrophy. Metabolic screening tests for Pompe disease, neurolipidosis, mucopolysaccharidosis, glycoproteinosis, mucolipidosis type I, and serum amino acids were normal.

The second patient, a 2-year-old sister of patient 1, with a height of 81 cm (Pc 10), weight of 11.2 kg (Pc 25), and occipitofrontal circumference (OCP) of 47 cm (Pc 25–50), presented moderately delayed psychomotor development (walked alone at 1.5 year old; had first syllables at 6 months without any progression afterward), micrognathia, and bilateral 2nd–3rd toes partial cutaneous syndactyly. Neurological examination showed gait disorders (an instable gait, with left lower limb rotated

Features	Patient 1	Patient 2	Patient 3
Neonatal hypotonia	+	+	+
Normal to accelerated growth	+	+	+
Absent to severely delayed speech	+	+	+
Global developmental delay	+	+	+
Minor dysmorphic facial features	+	+	+
Behavior characteristics			
• Autistic-like affect and behavior	+	+	+
• Mouthing or chewing nonfood items	—	—	—
• Decreased perception of pain	NA	NA	NA
Relatively large and fleshy hands	+	+	—
Dysplastic toenails	—	—	—
sacral dimple	+	—	—
Decreased perspiration	NA	NA	NA
Feeding difficulties	—	—	—
Strabismus	—	—	—
Renal problems	—	—	—
Seizures	—	—	—

NA, not assessed; +, present; –, absent.

Table 1.
Clinical characteristics of our patients.

outside) and speech delay (she says only few syllables). Psychiatric and psychologic evaluation revealed moderate developmental delay and autistic features (did not respond to commands; was not sociable, playing alone, and imitating only few actions). Her history included prolonged neonatal icterus (Crigler-Najjar syndrome type II). Her EEG was normal.

The third patient, an 11-year-old girl, presented delayed psychomotor development; she walked alone at 2 years and said first syllables after 5 years. The neurological evaluation at 11 years and 7 months showed severe intellectual disability and severe speech delay (she said only few mono- and disyllabic words, understood few simple orders). Brain MRI showed cerebellar subarachnoid cyst.

All three patients were investigated with genome-wide array CGH platforms. Array CGH experiments were performed using SurePrint G3 Human CGH Microarray Kits 180 K containing 170,334 distinct oligonucleotide probes (patients 1 and 2) and 60 k containing 55,077 distinct oligonucleotide probes (patient 3). The median probe spacing in RefSeq genes was 11 kb for 180 K platform and 33 kb for 60 K platform, respectively. The genomic gDNA was extracted using PureLink Genomic DNA Mini Kit (Invitrogen, Thermo Fisher Scientific); the concentration and quality of gDNA were assessed using a NanoDrop 2000 spectrophotometer (Thermo Fisher Scientific). Normal human gDNAs (*Agilent Human Reference DNA* Male or Female, according to the sex of the patient) were used as reference DNA. The experimental procedures were conducted using 1000 ng gDNA for 180 K microarray kit and 500 ng for 60 K microarray kit, for each sample (test and reference). After the enzymatic digestion of gDNA with *Alu*I and *Rsa*I, the reference DNA samples were labeled with cyanine 5-deoxyuridine triphosphate (Cy5-dUTP) and the patients DNA samples with Cy3-dUTP, respectively, using the

SureTag DNA Labeling Kit (Agilent Technologies). The labeled test and reference samples were pooled and purified together using Agilent Purification Columns. The DNA mixture was combined with Cot-1 DNA (Agilent Technologies), 10× aCGH blocking agent, and 2× HI-RPM hybridization buffer (Agilent Technologies); the mixture was dispensed to a microarray slide, assembled with an Agilent hybridization chamber, and incubated at 67°C for 24 h at 20 rpm. The hybridization was followed by a two-step washing procedure using Wash Buffer 1 and Wash Buffer 2 (Agilent Technologies). The microarray slides were scanned with Agilent SureScan Microarray Scanner system, and the data were extracted and analyzed using Agilent Cytogenomics software (Agilent Technologies). Copy number variations (CNVs) were called if they encompassed at least three consecutive probes with a log2 ratio value over 0.25 or below −0.25. For CNV clinical interpretation, public databases were used: UCSC (http://genome.ucsc.edu, accessed July 15, 2019); DGV (http://dgv.tcag.ca/dgv/app/), OMIM (http://www.omim.org/); DECIPHER (http://decipher.sanger.ac.uk/), and PubMed (https://www.ncbi.nlm.nih.gov/pubmed/).

3. Results and discussion

PMS has been under continuous investigation since its description [20, 21] that benefited, in many cases, by the strong cooperation of the PMS Foundation. Most of the patients were recruited in the USA [7, 12, 20–23] and Western Europe [9, 24–29]; there are also reports from Korea [30] and China [31]. PMS seems to be underdiagnosed in many parts of the world. However, the wide use of chromosomal microarray as a first-tier test for patients with neurodevelopmental disorders, autism, and congenital malformations [32] has greatly improved both diagnostic sensitivity and yield.

The array CGH results of our patients revealed deletions of 22q13 including SHANK3 gene. The genomic profiling of the two siblings (patients 1 and 2) revealed an identical 1.38 Mb interstitial duplication and a 1.565 Mb distal deletion: arr[GRCh37] 22q13.31q13.33(48202588_49585589)x3 and 22q13.33(49628598_51193680)x1 (**Figure 1a**). The deletion was confirmed by FISH. The duplication contained 2 miRNAs and *FAM19A5*, a gene coding a protein expressed mainly in the brain, considered a putative immunomodulator in nervous cells [5], while the 1.56 Mb deleted region included 37 genes, among which are *ALG12*, *MLC1*, *SBF1*, *SCO2*, *TYMP*, *MAPK8IP2*, *ARSA*, *SHANK3*, *ACR*, *TUBGCP6*, and *CHKB* (**Figure 1b**). Karyotype analysis and FISH testing of both parents (CTA799F10 probe, 22q13.33) showed no visible anomalies.

Patient 3 had a 3.514 Mb deletion, arr[GRCh37] 22q13.31q13.33 (47664025_51178264)x1, containing 41 genes, among which are *ALG12*, *MLC1*, *SBF1*, *SCO2*, *TYMP*, *MAPK8IP2*, *SHANK3*, *ARSA*, *TUBGCP6*, and *CHKB* (**Figure 2a** and **b**). The result was confirmed by FISH, using RP11-316I10 probe (22q11.21) and cosmide n85a3 (22q13.33).

The cytogenetic findings in PMS may be variable. In a study gathering 201 PMS patients analyzed by array CGH, the vast majority had 22q13 terminal deletions. Duplications, varying in size from 0.02 to 6.84 Mb, localized centromeric to the deleted region were detected in 9% of patients [7]. Two of our patients (patients 1 and 2, siblings) have a similar pattern and a proximal duplication that accompanies a terminal deletion. This type of duplication-deletion cytogenetic changes have been reported for many chromosomes, and it is most likely mediated by a U-type exchange between sister chromatids [33]. Patient 3 had a simple terminal deletion.

22q13 region in the vicinity of SHANK3 gene is rich in genes with a high expression in the brain and also a high probability of *loss of function intolerance* [19, 34].

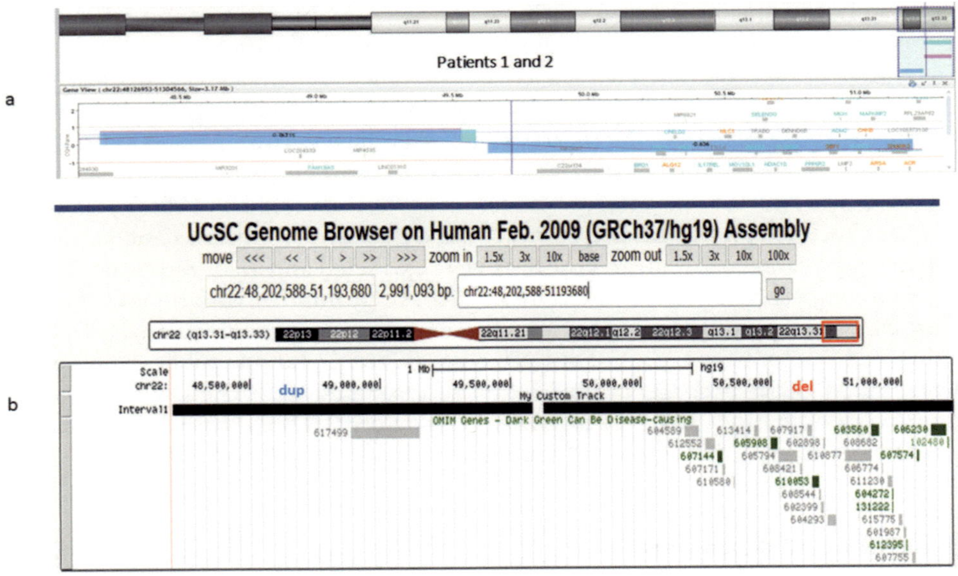

Figure 1.
(a) The genomic profiling of the two siblings (patients 1 and 2) revealing an identical 1.38 Mb interstitial duplication and a 1.565 Mb distal deletion and (b) UCSC Genome Browser window showing the genomic coordinates of the detected variants.

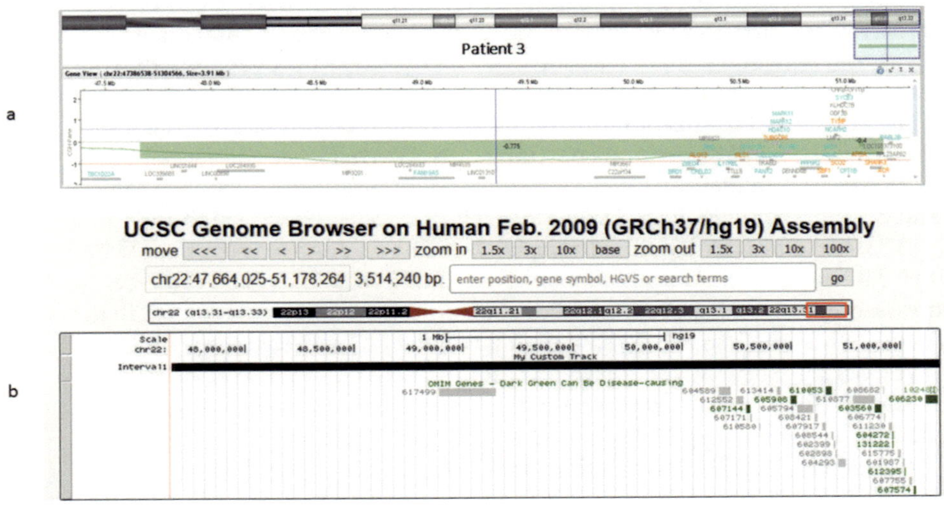

Figure 2.
(a) The genomic profiling of the patient 3 showing a 3.514 Mb deletion and (b) UCSC Genome Browser window showing the genomic coordinates of the detected variant.

The haploinsufficiency of these genes is considered to contribute not only to the variability of the phenotype but also to the neuropsychiatric features of PMS.

Among the genes located on 22q, *PARVB* and *SULT4A1* genes (telomeric to *SHANK3*) have been associated with increased severity of PMS [29]. Mitogen-activated protein kinase 8-interacting protein 2 (*MAPK8IP2*) localized centromeric to *SHANK3* codes a protein with high expressivity in the brain (postsynaptic density); experimental animal studies showed that mice lacking *MAPK8IP2* had motor and cognitive deficits [35]. *MLC1* gene variants have been reported as causal for megalencephalic leukoencephalopathy characterized by regression of development. Taking into account the prevalence of regression symptoms in PMS, the relation between deletion of *MLC1* gene and regression might bring new insights [35].

Other genes in this region have been involved in particular aspects of PMS (e.g., *NUP50*, *CERK*, *KIAA1644*, *PHF21B*, *c22orf9*, *FBLN1*, *CELSR1*, or miRNA molecules located at 22q) [7]. Frye et al. [36] brought evidence that haploinsufficiency of genes related to mitochondrial functioning, located at or close to 22q13.3 (e.g., *TRMU*, *SCO2*, *TYMP*, *CPT1B*), may explain a part of the phenotypic variation in PMS patients.

PARVB and *WNT7B* gene loss as well as larger or more proximal deletions of 22q have been associated with absent speech [5, 7]. In addition, Soorya et al. [10] reported in 2013 that expressive and receptive language skills were not significantly associated with deletion size. Our patients 1 and 3 had absent speech; patient 2, evaluated at 2 years of age, also presented speech delay. The regions deleted in our patients did not correlate with the abovementioned genetic regions nor include *PARVB* and *WNT7B* genes. However, both of our patients exhibited ASD, which has been associated with smaller deleted segments [5]. Aggressive behavior, present in patient 1, has been assumed to be inversely correlated with the deletion size [7]. Brain structural anomalies, among which is corpus callosum hypoplasia, are reported in the literature to be present in 25–66% of patients [5]; this anomaly was present also in the first patient. Patient 3 has a cerebellar subarachnoid cyst, also reported in PMS patients [4]. Patient 2 did not undergo brain MRI.

4. Conclusion

PMS is a rare disorder, with a broad phenotypic spectrum, which often goes underdiagnosed. Although the phenotype is clinically heterogeneous, PMS should be considered in any patient with global developmental delay, absent or severely delayed speech, and autistic behavior, in association with some minor dysmorphic features (dolichocephaly, ear anomalies, periorbital fullness, epicanthal folds, hypertelorism, long eyelashes, bulbous nose, pointed chin, large fleshy hands) and hypotonia. The most common medical complications include seizures, gastrointestinal problems, renal anomalies, and respiratory infections [4]. Brain MRI images showed a high prevalence of arachnoid cysts, ventriculomegaly, dysmyelination, and morphological changes of the corpus callosum [4]. Clinical practice parameters reviewed by Kolevzon et al. [4] aimed to provide guidelines for evaluation and monitoring. The clinical evaluation and regular monitoring of patients with PMS should include psychiatric, psychological, neurologic, endocrinological, cardiologic, gastroenterological, nephrological, and pediatric examinations. After a review of all case series reported previously, the authors concluded that there are no specific features for the syndrome and the diagnosis of PMS is genetic [4]. Recommended genetic tests are chromosomal microarray (as a first-tier test), MLPA, and FISH; if these tests are not informative in a patient, mutations should be searched by NGS or Sanger sequencing.

Regarding the therapeutic strategy, patients can benefit from early intervention targeted to improve their muscle strength and communication abilities, including physical, speech, occupational, and behavioral therapies [1]. There are very few studies on different medications in patients with PMS [37]. One study investigated the effect of intranasal insulin—six individuals with PMS received 0.5–1.5 IU/day three times daily for 12 months, with good effects both on motor development and cognitive functions [38]. In another study on 25 children with PMS, intranasal insulin improved intellectual and behavioral development, especially in children older than 3 years, but most results were not statistically significant (Netherlands

Trial Registry ID: NTR3758). Studies on mice and human neuronal models brought evidence that insulin-like growth factor-1 (IGF-1) reverts synaptic deficits in PMS [4, 27], as well as in Rett syndrome [4, 27], most probably due to its positive effects on synaptic development, neurogenesis, and brain vessel growth [27]. Clinical studies with IGF-1 and related compounds in autism spectrum disorders, including PMS, are ongoing.

PMS is a rare disorder with a wide phenotypic spectrum and a large genomic landscape. *SHANK3* gene is considered the main culprit for the neuropsychiatric phenotype; however, its role must be investigated in the broader genetic landscape. Insights into the contribution of other genes at 22q13 are gained from genomic profiling, leading to refined genotype-phenotype correlations. PMS clinical diagnosis is challenging, as no pathognomonic features are described. Intellectual disability/global developmental delay, severe speech impairment, autistic features, motor impairments, and mild dysmorphic traits stand as the main clinical characteristics.

Genetic diagnosis of PMS has greatly benefited from the introduction of chromosomal microarray. As no characteristic clinical features are described, genomic profiling by microarray as a first-tier approach drives the diagnosis. Furthermore, the detailed molecular characterization has advanced the understanding of different gene contributions to PMS pathogenesis, thus paving the way for identification of therapeutic targets.

Acknowledgements

BAC probes RP11-316I10 (22q11.21), CTA799F10, and cosmid n85a3 (22q13.33) were kindly provided by Professor Jean-Michel Dupont, Laboratoire de Cytogénétique, APHP, HUPC-Site Cochin, Paris, France.

Ethics

Written consent forms, for research and publishing the data of the patients, were obtained from the parents.

Funding

The work was partially supported by the Ministry of Research and Innovation in Romania, under Program 1 – The Improvement of the National System of Research and Development, Subprogram 1.2 – Institutional Excellence – Projects of Excellence Funding in RDI, Contract No. 7PFE/16.10.2018 and Core Program Grants PN 09.33.02.03, PN 16.22.05.01.

Author details

Magdalena Budisteanu[1,2,3†], Andreea Tutulan-Cunita[1,5†], Ina Ofelia Focsa[1,4], Sorina Mihaela Papuc[1] and Aurora Arghir[1,4*]

1 "Victor Babes" National Institute of Pathology, Bucharest, Romania

2 "Prof. Dr. Alex. Obregia" Clinical Hospital of Psychiatry, Bucharest, Romania

3 "Titu Maiorescu" University, Bucharest, Romania

4 "Carol Davila" University of Medicine and Pharmacy, Bucharest, Romania

5 Cytogenomic Medical Laboratory, Bucharest, Romania

*Address all correspondence to: aurora.arghir@ivb.ro

† These authors contributed equally.

References

[1] Phelan MC. Deletion 22q13.3 syndrome. Orphanet Journal of Rare Diseases. 2008;**3**:14-19

[2] Phelan K, McDermid HE. The 22q13.3 deletion syndrome (Phelan-McDermid syndrome). Molecular Syndromology. 2012;**2**:186-201

[3] Zwanenburg RJ, Bocca G, Ruiter SAJ, Dilingh JH, Flapper BCT, van den Heuvel ER, et al. Is there an effect of intranasal insulin on development and behaviour in Phelan-McDermid syndrome? A randomized, double-blind, placebo-controlled trial. European Journal of Human Genetics. 2016;**24**:1696-1701

[4] Kolevzon A, Angarita B, Bush L, Wang AT, Franck Y, Yang A, et al. Phelan-McDermid syndrome: A review of the literature and practice parameters for medical assessment and monitoring. Journal of Neurodevelopmental Disorders. 2014;**6**:39-50

[5] Tabet AC, Roland T, Ducloy M, Lévy J, Buratti J, Mathieu A, et al. A framework to identify modifier genes in patients with Phelan-McDermid syndrome. NPJ Genomic Medicine. 2017;**2**:32

[6] Phelan K, Rogers RC, Boccuto L. Phelan-McDermid Syndrome. In: Adam MP, Ardinger HH, Pagon RA, et al., editors. GeneReviews® [Internet]. Seattle, WA: University of Washington, Seattle; 1993-2019. 2005. Available from: https://www.ncbi.nlm.nih.gov/books/NBK1198/

[7] Sarasua SM, Boccuto L, Sharp JL, Dwivedi A, Chen CF, Rollins JD, et al. Clinical and genomic evaluation of 201 patients with Phelan-McDermid syndrome. Human Genetics. 2014;**133**:847-859

[8] Anderlid BM, Schoumans J, Anneren G, Tapia-Paez I, Dumanski J, Blennow E, et al. FISH-mapping of a 100-kb terminal 22q13 deletion. Human Genetics. 2002;**110**:439-443

[9] Bonaglia MC, Giorda R, Mani E, Aceti G, Anderlid B-M, Baroncini A, et al. Identification of a recurrent breakpoint within the *SHANK3* gene in the 22q13.3 deletion syndrome. Journal of Medical Genetics. 2006;**43**:822-828

[10] Soorya L, Kolevzon A, Zweifach J, Lim T, Dobry Y, Schwartz L, et al. Prospective investigation of autism and genotype-phenotype correlations in 22q13 deletion syndrome and SHANK3 deficiency. Molecular Autism. 2013;**4**(1):18

[11] Boccuto L, Lauri M, Sarasua SM, Skinner CD, Buccella D, Dwivedi A, et al. Prevalence of SHANK3 variants in patients with different subtypes of autism spectrum disorders. European Journal of Human Genetics. 2013;**21**:310-316

[12] Sarasua SM, Dwivedi A, Boccuto L, Chen CF, Sharp JL, Rollins JD, et al. 22q13.2q13.32 genomic regions associated with severity of speech delay, developmental delay, and physical features in Phelan-McDermid syndrome. Genetics in Medicine. 2014;**16**(4):318-328

[13] Phelan K, Boccuto L, Rogers RC, Sarasua SM, McDermid HE. Letter to the editor regarding Disciglio et al.: Interstitial 22q13 deletions not involving *SHANK3* gene: A new contiguous gene syndrome. American Journal of Medical Genetics—Part A. 2015;**167A**:1679-1680

[14] Wilson HL, Crolla JA, Walker D, Artifoni L, Dallapiccola B, Takano T, et al. Interstitial 22q13 deletions: Genes

other than SHANK3 have major effects on cognitive and language development. European Journal of Human Genetics. 2008;**16**(11):1301-1310

[15] Darnell JC. Defects in translational regulation contributing to human cognitive and behavioral disease. Current Opinion in Genetics & Development. 2011;**21**(4):465-473

[16] Sakai Y, Shaw CA, Dawson BC, Dugas DV, Al-Mohtaseb Z, Hill DE, et al. Protein interactome reveals converging molecular pathways among autism disorders. Science Translational Medicine. 2011;**3**(86):86ra49

[17] Shcheglovitov A, Shcheglovitov O, Yazawa M, Portmann T, Shu R, Sebastiano V, et al. SHANK3 and IGF1 restore synaptic deficits in neurons from 22q13 deletion syndrome patients. Nature. 2013;**503**:267-271

[18] Yi F, Danko T, Botelho SC, Patzke C, Pak CH, Wernig M, et al. Autism-associated SHANK3 haploinsufficiency causes I_h channelopathy in human neurons. Science. 2016;**352**(6286):aaf2669

[19] Mitz AR, Philyaw TJ, Boccuto L, Shcheglovitov A, Sarasua SM, Kaufmann WE, et al. Identification of 22q13 genes most likely to contribute to Phelan McDermid syndrome. European Journal of Human Genetics. 2018;**26**:293-302

[20] Flint J, Wilkie AOM, Buckle VJ, Winter RB, Holland AJ, McDermid HE. The detection of subtelomericchromosomalrearrangements in idiopathic mental retardation. Nature Genetics. 1995;**9**:132-139

[21] Phelan MC, Rogers RC, Saul RA, Stapleton GA, Sweet K, McDermid H, et al. 22q13 deletion syndrome. American Journal of Medical Genetics. 2001;**101**:91-99

[22] Dhar SU, del Gaudio D, German JR, Peters SU, Ou Z, Bader PI, et al. 22q13.3 deletion syndrome: Clinical and molecular analysis using array CGH. American Journal of Medical Genetics. Part A. 2010;**152A**(3):573-581

[23] Bro D, O'Hara R, Primeau M, Hanson-Kahn A, Hallmayer J, Bernstein JA. Sleep disturbances in individuals with Phelan-McDermid syndrome: Correlation with caregivers' sleep quality and daytime functioning. Sleep. 2017;**40**(2):zsw062

[24] Bonaglia MC, Giorda R, Beri S, De Agostini C, Novara F, Fichera M, et al. Molecular mechanisms generating and stabilizing terminal 22q13 deletions in 44 subjects with Phelan/McDermid syndrome. PLoS Genetics. 2011;**7**(7):e1002173

[25] Denayer A, Van Esch H, de Ravel T, Frijns JP, Van Buggenhout G, Vogels A, et al. Neuropsychopathology in 7 patients with the 22q13 deletion syndrome: Presence of bipolar disorder and progressive loss of skills. Molecular Syndromology. 2012;**3**(1):14-20

[26] Verhoeven WMA, Egger JIM, Cohen-Snuijf R, Kant SG, de Leeuw N. Phelan-Mcdermid syndrome: Clinical report of a 70-year-old woman. American Journal of Medical Genetics—Part A. 2013;**161A**:158-161

[27] Kolevzon A, Bush L, Wang AT, Halpern D, Frank Y, Grodberg D, et al. A pilot controlled trial of insulin-like growth factor-1 in children with Phelan-McDermid syndrome. Molecular Autism. 2014;**5**:54-62

[28] Egger JIM, Zwanenburg RJ, van Ravenswaaij-Arts CMA, Kleefstra T, Verhoeven WMA. Neuropsychological phenotype and psychopathology in seven adult patients with Phelan-McDermid syndrome: Implications for treatment strategy. Genes, Brain, and Behavior. 2016;**15**:395-404

[29] Zwanenburg RJ, Ruiter SAJ, van den Heuvel ER, Flapper BCT, Van Ravenswaaij-Ars CMA. Developmental phenotype in Phelan McDermid (22q13.2 deletion) syndrome: A systematic and prospective study in 34 children. Journal of Neurodevelopmental Disorders. 2016;**8**:16-27

[30] Kim YM, Choi IH, Kim JS, Kim JH, Cho JH, Lee BH, et al. Phelan-McDermid syndrome presenting with developmental delays and facial dysmorphisms. Korean Journal of Pediatrics. 2016;**59**(Suppl 1):S25-S28

[31] Lei D, Li S, Banerjee S, Zhang H, Li C, Hou S, et al. Clinical and genomic evaluation of a Chinese patient with a novel deletion associated with Phelan-McDermid syndrome. Oncotarget. 2016;**7**(49):80327-80335

[32] Miller DT, Adam MP, Aradhya S, Biesecker LG, Brothman AR, Carter NP, et al. Consensus statement: Chromosomal microarray is a first-tier clinical diagnostic test for individuals with developmental disabilities or congenital anomalies. American Journal of Human Genetics. 2010;**86**(5):749-764

[33] Rowe LR, Lee J, Rector L, Kaminsky EB, Brothman AR, Martin CL, et al. U-type exchange is the most frequent mechanism for inverted duplication with terminal deletion rearrangements. Journal of Medical Genetics. 2009;**46**:694-702

[34] Lek M, Karczewski KJ, Minikel EV, Samocha KE, Banks E, Fennell T, et al. Analysis of protein-coding genetic variation in 60,706 humans. Nature. 2016;**536**(7616):285-291

[35] Ziats CA, Grosvenor LP, Sarasua SM, Thurm AE, Swedo SE, Mahfouz A, et al. Functional genomics analysis of Phelan-McDermid syndrome 22q13 region during human neurodevelopment. PLoS ONE. 2019;**14**(3):e0213921

[36] Frye RE, Cox D, Slattery J, Tippett M, Kahler S, Granpeesheh D, et al. Mitochondrial dysfunction may explain symptom variation in Phelan-McDermid syndrome. Scientific Reports. 2015;**6**:19544

[37] Costales JL, Kolevzon A. Phelan-McDermid syndrome and SHANK3: Implications for treatment. Neurotherapeutics. 2015;**12**:620-630

[38] Schmidt H, Kern W, Giese R, Hallschmid M, Enders A. Intranasal insulin to improve developmental delay in children with 22q13 deletion syndrome: An exploratory clinical trial. Journal of Medical Genetics. 2009;**46**:217-222

Chapter 7

The Energy as a Determinant Factor in the Ethiopathogeny of Chromosomal Abnormalities. The Unsuspected Bioenergetic Role of Melanin

Arturo Solis Herrera

Abstract

In the study of chromosomal abnormalities, in genetics, and in medicine in general, attention is rarely paid to the role of energy in the healthy subject and in the sick patient. The research on the chromosomal anomalies that are constantly published, does not mention the energy necessary for the biochemical processes involved in the function, replication and formation of genes, to be carried out in an adequate way. It seems that it is assumed that energy levels are always fine or at least did not have a significant role in the conditions associated with what we call chromosomal anomalies. A characteristic of the cell nucleus that has gone unnoticed is that it contains neither mitochondria nor ATP, much less glucose. Perhaps because of this, some researchers and clinicians come to think that the nucleus of cells does not require energy. The purpose of this work is to draw attention to the importance of energy levels in all the metabolic processes of the cell; and to make known that glucose is not an energy source, as it is only a source of carbon chains; and finally remark that our body, through melanin, can take energy directly from light.

Keywords: melanin, water dissociation, energy, hydrogen, aneuploidy

1. Background

Diseases attributed to chromosomal abnormalities are currently perceived as a defect occurring at the deepest level of mutations in the complex sequence of nucleic acids and causing biochemical, clinical or physical manifestations. The so-called genetic diseases do not have yet a specific treatment, at most only symptomatic; because the problem has proved more complex than anticipated, as gene therapy in its diverse form has not yielded the expected results; therefore alterations in the bases, or in genes, or in chromosomes, or inclusive in histones have been more extensive and complicated than expected.

The chromosome is called the highly organized structures, made up of DNA and proteins, which contains most of the genetic information of a living being. The DNA double helix is bound to proteins called histones. The histones have positively charged (basic) amino acids to bind the negatively charged (acidic) DNA. The DNA is wrapped around the histone core of eight protein subunits, forming the nucleosome. The nucleosome is clamped by histone H1. About 200 base pairs (bp) of DNA coil around one histone [1].

Methylation of histone or of DNA usually turns a gene off. Acetylation of histone usually turns a gene on. Phosphorylation is not known what that does. The only thing they have in common is that for them to happen properly, they require energy, and in various ways, not just activation energy.

Prokaryotic cells (bacteria) contain their chromosome as circular DNA. Usually, the entire genome is a single circle, but often there are extra circles called plasmids. The DNA is packaged by DNA-binding proteins.

The bacterial DNA is packaged in loops back and forth. The bundled DNA is called the nucleoid. It concentrates the DNA in part of the cell, but it is not separated by a nuclear membrane (as in eukaryotes). The DNA does form loops back and forth to a protein core, attached to the cell wall [2]. By the way, melanin, in prokaryotics, is in the cell wall mainly.

Chromosomes are fundamental part of genetic information, comprising molecular DNA wrapped in a highly complex form by histones that surround the double helix. Damage or even minute changes to the structure of the chromosomes, genes, nucleotides or histones can lead to diverse health problems and health defects. Having too many or too few chromosomes in a cell can be considered as chromosomal abnormality.

Chromosome abnormalities, even to the nucleotide level, may cast light on the nature of mechanisms whereby normal anatomy evolves, and abnormal anatomy arises. Correlating genotype to phenotype is a formidable challenge exercise [3].

The number of chromosomes, as well as every one of the structures that make up them is astonishingly accurate and is repeated every day from the beginning of time. Then, why are the alterations to whether is in genes or chromosomes? And even more, why are chromosomal alterations not isolated or unique? If the energy source is ATP and therefore mitochondria, why does the cell nucleus have none?

2. Introduction

The chromosome is the heart of a central paradox in evolution. How do species in the three kingdoms remain the same over long periods of geological time and generate enough variability to produce new species, sometimes relatively rapid? [4]. Stability versus change is a crucial dichotomy in molecular biology. The events that bring about stability and change in DNA structure involve processes of replication, transcription and recombination; and since beginning of time, similar mechanisms operate in the three living kingdoms.

Free living bacteria need genetic information and energy to synthesize proteins that means energy expenditure for executing vital functions. Most bacteria have a single chromosome with DNA that is about 2 Mbp (mega base pairs) long (1 Mbp = 1,000,000 base pairs), being the DNA content of different species variable from 0.58 to greater than 9 Mbp of DNA, and some bacteria have multiple chromosomes.

3. Energy and chromosomes

Eukaryotic organisms generally have larger chromosomes than bacteria. In humans, the 5000 Mbp of haploid DNA is distributed among 22 autosomes and 2 sex-specific chromosomes. Larger chromosomes mean more energy expenditure in many ways. Eukaryotic DNA is in a compartment, the nucleus, which is separated by a phospholipid-containing membrane from cytoplasmic ribosomes and protein translation activity. Cell uses energy in many ways, even to keep the shape, the organization, function, compartmentalization, etc. During cell division, the eukaryotic nuclear membrane breaks down once per cell cycle to distribute the 46 diploid chromosomes equally between 2 daughter cells. We must keep in mind, that any change requires energy, so, every step during cell division need energy to happen, and the amount and type of energy must be same as has been since the beginning of time.

Eukaryotic genomes must be condensed by several orders of magnitude to fit in the largest cell organelle: the nucleus. Compaction of genomes is achieved by coiling the DNA around histone proteins to form a chromatin fiber, which is subsequently folded into complex higher order structures such as loops, domains and compartments [5]. The coiling of DNA and subsequent folding requires energy.

Despite the ubiquitous presence of all major architectural features of genomes, there is considerable variability and heterogeneity in genome organization at the single-cell level [6]. Although the position of chromosomes and genes are non-random in the cell population, their patterns of location are variable among individual cells [7]. This variable location probably has relationship with the concept that every melanosome is unique.

The fundamental variability of genome organization is mirrored by stochasticity in the transcription process itself [8]. Active transcription generally occurs in short bursts at irregular intervals [9], requiring energy in several ways. This pattern of punctuated gene transcription is common to all organisms, particularly widespread in mammals [10]. There is a dynamic binding of transcription factors and chromatin motion [11], requiring both energy expenditure.

The stochastic nature of transcription points to structural heterogeneity of the chromatin fiber and of the genome as a whole, thereby energy requirements must be conceptualized with the same characteristics, as a whole (**Figure 1**).

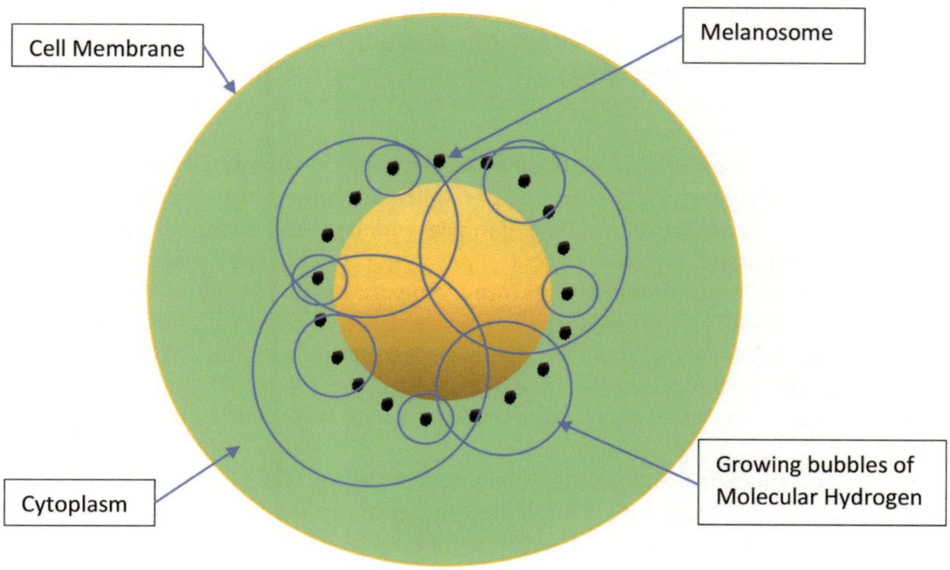

Figure 1.
Diagram to show the organization of melanosomes located in the perinuclear space, forming full envelopment around the cell nucleus. Melanin releases molecular hydrogen (H_2) and molecular oxygen (O_2) symmetrically, in all directions, following the laws of simple diffusion; like growing spheres of energy. These energy bubbles coalescing forming high energy areas inside and outside cell nucleus. These facts explain the energy for the cell nucleus, a zone of high energy expenditure, in absence of ATP and mitochondria.

The large-scale genome structures, such as chromatin compartments, are consistently present in individual cells, but smaller organizational units, such as chromatin domains, are variable between cells [12]. This is congruous with the concept that any melanosome is unique.

The stochasticity observed in gene expression is indeed paralleled by high variability in genome organization [13]. Therefore, although chromatin domains can be observed in individual cells, their boundaries are highly variable. The relative position of individual chromatin domains within compartments varies considerably, and modeling suggest dynamic movement within individual chromatin domains [14], this dynamic movement requires energy.

Looping events are highly variable between cells and are likely to be dynamic (energy expenditure), forming and reforming many times during a single interphase [15]. The cell uses energy in many ways and at the same time, for instance, regulate chromatin loop stability and loop formation, this is a different processes with apparently distinct dynamics that are regulated and impelled when it is necessary with the same energy.

Interestingly, the behavior of the two alleles in the same nucleus is not correlated, which suggests that the variability present is largely intrinsic and not dependent on cell-level variables such as cycle stage [16]. However, energy was not considered as a variable by the authors.

The observations are consistent with a single-cell mapping data showing that individual interactions underlying the formation of chromatin domains and loops are highly variable [17]. By the way, any interaction requires available energy.

Thereby, several observations demonstrate a high degree of heterogeneity in genome organization, suggesting that in individual cells in a population, genomes can assume distinct, albeit related; spatial conformations mediated by short-lived chromatin-chromatin interactions rather than by persistent or pervasive associations. This complex variability does not imply that structural features of chromatin organization are not relevant for gene functions, but rather it suggests that structural heterogeneity may be another layer modulating the stochasticity of gene expression [18]. We must keep in mind that any change requires energy, therefore chromatin organization and gene expression need energy in several, accurate and distinct ways.

Genome organization is a highly complex issue but at the same time is intrinsically flexible and is so strict in terms of energy requirements; furthermore, the two alleles in a cell may be differentially organized which means energy expenditure with a highly accuracy. Genes such as the permanently inactive immunoglobulin loci, as well as the entire inactive X chromosome are located at the nuclear periphery, which are zones of low energy; whereas their active counterparts are found nearer the center of the nucleus [19] that is a high energy zone due to confluence of growing bubbles of molecular hydrogen (H_2) coming from the melanosomes (**Figure 2**) that completely surround the nucleus located mainly in the perinuclear space.

In olfactory neurons, thousands of olfactory receptor (OR) loci that are not expressed are sequestered into a single heterochromatin focus [20]. Thereby, the genome organization and its stochastic nature may be a universal mechanism in establishing differences in the cellular properties of alleles [21], that in turn requires universal energy.

There is little correlation between interactions of the two alleles of the same cell. The allele-specific mapping data demonstrate that the two alleles in a cell generally contact different sets of partners [22]. This contact and relative processes undoubtedly require energy.

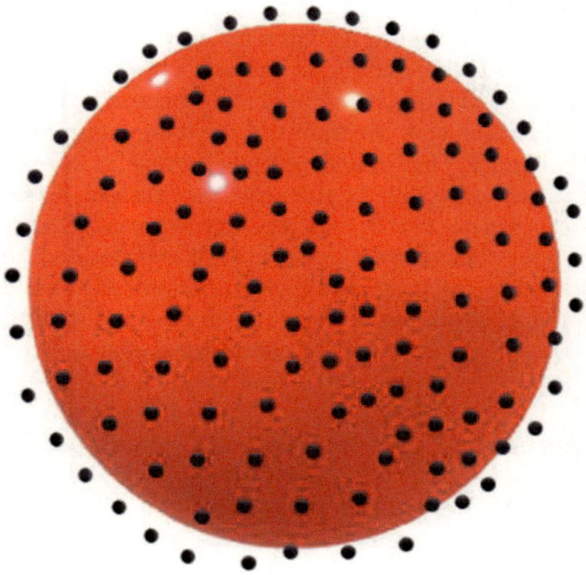

Figure 2.
The main location of melanosomes is in the perinuclear space, covering the entire cell nucleus surface.

The range of distance by most locus pair is roughly 1-μm radius of constraint typically observed for DNA movement in live cells, and long-range events are rare [23], but as small as they are, such movements require energy.

The interaction of chromatin proteins with their substrate is dynamic, even for the architectural proteins that forms "stable" loops, such as CTCF and cohesin [24]. It takes energy both for chromatin proteins to interact with their substrate, as well as to preserve form.

In transgenic systems in *Drosophilia*, colocalization between promoter and their cognate enhancers is necessary for proper expression in cis and trans [25], which also requires the use of adequate energy. It appears that the movement of enhancer elements, as well as their position relative to promoters, is functionally relevant. Again, any movement, any change; requires energy with no exception.

Cancer-relevant translocations occur more frequently among chromosomes that are in spatial proximity, which suggests that variability in spatial organization strongly determines the repertoire of translocations in a given cell type or tissue [26], which means that normal spatial organization requires normal generation and distribution of energy (from melanin).

In some cases, active loci move less than silenced ones [27], whereas, for other genes, actively transcribing alleles show increased mobility [28]. Energy is involved in both cases, indeed.

Furthermore, haploinsufficiency, mutation and down regulation of the architectural protein CTCF, all of which lead to destabilization of chromatin loops and cause more variability in genome organization, have tumor-promoting effects including deregulation of cancer-relevant gene expression programs, disruption of cell polarity and a decrease in patient survival [29]. Cell polarity and all above-cited processes require energy.

It is a long-lasting observation that a cancer cell has a low voltage, which is congruous with low levels of energy that is also consistent with the observation of extensive heterogeneity in tumors [30].

The generation of a stable output from variable inputs is a complex challenge. The extensive structural heterogeneity in genome organization on the one hand,

and on the other hand, the requirement for establishment and maintenance of stable cells states means that the energy from melanin is a major driver in gene expression and genome function, acting as intrinsic noise present in individual cells.

The purpose of the description of some of the processes that happen at the nucleus was to highlight the very accurate and constant energy they require to happen in a timely manner. The generation and distribution of energy, from melanin, is an exact, that when we alter its anatomy, for example, by sectioning the cell membrane, the process is noticeably disturbed and stopped. Hence, the impossibility of properly studying the vital processes happens constantly in the living cell.

Cell nucleus activity is constant, as it happens incessantly both day and night, and cannot be explained based on the dogma of glucose and ATP as energy sources; because the cell nucleus normally does not contain either.

4. Enzymes require energy (from melanin) to carry out its function

The complexity of chromosomes biology can be represented by the enzymes that explain the untangling enigma are topoisomerases, which break and rejoin DNA molecules; allowing individual strands to pass one through another. These enzymes have, at least; two important roles: they provide a swivel to allow processes such as replication and transcription to proceed unimpeded, and they untangle knots and inter-chromosome links between DNA molecules [31].

The phosphodiester bonds that are broken and reformed per reaction cycles [32] require the presence of available energy, however, cell nucleus has neither ATP nor mitochondria. Furthermore, chromatin (DNA + proteins attached to a chromosome) must be folded many times to fit within a cell nucleus; and the highly accurate processes of folding and unfolding also requires energy.

In all organisms, DNA becomes organized in turns of the double strand over the interwound twists of the Watson-Crick helix, named supercoils or σ which represents the number of super-helical turns divided by the Watson-Crick turns of a double helix. The formation and maintenance of this highly complex organized structure requires energy. Supercoiling influences the Watson-Crick structure and, like the spring, the mechanical energy of super negative coils or opposite to the handedness of the Watson-Crick turns; increases exponentially with quantity [33]. However, this kind of energy (mechanical) does not have the properties of accuracy, direction and force that could explain the extraordinary characteristics and dynamics of folded DNA structures.

In the average eukaryotic nucleus, nuclear DNA is several times more concentrated than bacterial DNA. Eukaryotic DNA is wrapped tightly around nucleosomes, generating solenoidal supercoils that condense DNA 8-fold [34], which means significant energy expenditure.

DNA is a plectonemic helix [31], this is two helical strands entwine around each other (**Figure 3**). Two antiparallel strands of DNA are interwound once for every 10 base pairs. Because of this wound configuration, biochemical transactions that involve strand separation require chromosome movement (spin) about DNA's long axis. The processes of DNA replication, recombination and transcription all require DNA rotation, and during DNA synthesis the rotation speed approaches 6000 rpm. This amazing rotation speed indeed requires energy, as any one of the biochemical transactions involved. The question remains: Where come from the energy for the cell nucleus? There is neither mitochondria nor ATP.

Supercoiled branches are dynamic so that opposing DNA in one supercoiling domain interact more than 100 times more frequently with other proteins in the same domain than it does with other proteins bound to a different domain. These biochemical processes are astonishing accurate, they do not happen by chance, and those rates of domain interactions requires energy in many ways [35].

In the eukaryotic nucleus, enzymes such as RNA polymerase gain access to DNA, which remains histone bound throughout most biochemical transactions. There are complex interactions that require energy in continuous an adequate form. The way in which multiple proteins interact with coated DNA nucleosomes is not completely understood but it is for sure that requires energy.

When DNA is liberated from cells by breaking the peptidoglycan coat, chromosomes form bundled loops that represent domains. Such preparations (called nucleoids) behave as discrete bodies [36]. Every step above described requires energy, which must be in a very precise location, amount, availability and quality. By the way, energy is defined as everything that produces a change.

Many reactions of the chromosome require the formation of intricate DNA-protein machines to replicate, transcribe or recombine DNA at specific sequences. Thereby, many reactions mean substantive energy expenditure. Chromosome-associated proteins assist in the formation of complexes by shaping DNA that include HU, H-NS, integration host factor (IHF) and factor for inversion stimulation (FIS) [37]. These highly complex and accurate processes need energy in many ways. For instance, proteins tend to dissolve in aqueous media thereby energy is required to keep the shape, not only to carry out their function.

In addition to the histones, eukaryotic chromosomes contain regulatory proteins that are much less abundant. One class of proteins, the high mobility group (HMG) family of DNA-binding proteins, bends DNA much like bacterial proteins IHF and FIS [38].

Any chemical process requires activation energy to happen, but the amount and type of energy must be accurate in location, quantity and quality, otherwise it does not happen, or at least will occurs differently, or perhaps happens in excess, and there would be significant variations in quantity and nature of the reaction products, which is non-compatible with the highly accuracy of life's biochemical processes.

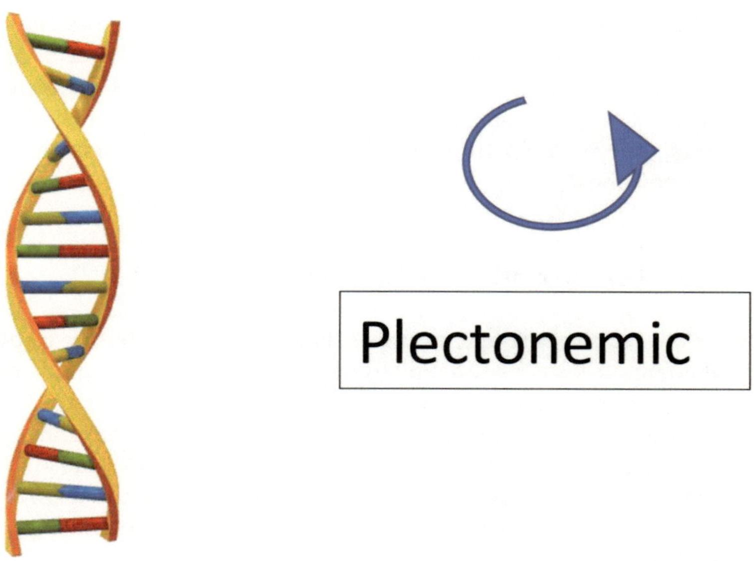

Figure 3.
DNA is plectonemic [31] and keeping chromosomes untangled requires a special class of enzymes called topoisomerases, however, both chromosomes and enzymes requires energy to function properly.

5. Genetic therapies failures

Those who are engaged in the understanding and therapy of genetic disorders are aware that common single-nucleotide polymorphisms may be strongly associated with an outcome (based on highly significant *P* values) and yet have very modest effect sizes (based on the odds ratios) thereby, it have been recognized that if there are differences in the genetic characteristics associated with the initiation of a disease versus its progression (presumably representing the outcomes of different biological pathways), we may have to tailor therapies (and their timing) to address these different stages of disease, for instance, antisense oligonucleotides [39].

Thus, pharmacologic targets based on abnormal genes may have clinical relevance for treating the progression of these conditions as well. However, the failure of clinical trials based on this kind of therapy apparently rational is the rule. Perhaps, measuring the effectiveness of this therapeutic approach by measuring the rates of progression of genetic diseases may not only fail but also mislead us from recognizing potential benefits at early stages of the disease [40].

It is possible to use the genetic endophenotypes [41], of these individuals conduct clinical trials that can address the inhibition of disease initiation and/or slow the disease progression prior to the development of overt systemic symptoms and advanced somatic findings.

Since 1949, Linus Pauling published about molecular diseases [42] and chromosomes are constituted by molecules. However, in biology, nothing has sense except at light of evolution, and chromosomes cannot explain the origin of life, thereby what's behind the chromosomes? What gave rise to genes? What causes atoms to sort in a certain way and conform to complex organic molecules? We think the mysterious force behind these questions all is energy.

But it is not any kind of energy, it is a very special energy that is precise, adequate, constant and which is constantly available. Such an astonishingly accurate type of energy, as nature wastes nothing, it cannot come from the oxidation of glucose or from the hydrolysis of ATP in ADP.

We believe that the energy that directs the formation of the molecules that make up the chromosomes, as well as their proper functioning and even their replication is the energy that comes from sunlight, but must be transformed into chemical energy by dissociating water molecule to make it wearable, such as chlorophyll in plants. Our discovery of melanin's unsuspected intrinsic ability to transform sunlight into chemical energy, by dissociating the molecule from water, such as chlorophyll in plants, will mark a before and after in biology, and even more so in the biology of chromosomes.

6. Chromosomal abnormalities in the oocytes

The oocyte is a relatively simple example that allows us to observe important chromosomal anomalies, such as aneuploidy. The oocyte has been and is highly studied because female fertility declines dramatically depending on age [43]. Arrested human embryos are more likely to have abnormal chromosomes than developing embryos from women of advanced maternal age [44]. Most arrested embryos have multiple chromosome anomalies, indicating that the factors causing aneuploidy may also affect embryo development. The detailed relationship between embryo development and aneuploidy is not known.

Chromosomal anomalies could occur in any chromosome, and the proportion of anomalies in the most common 5 chromosomes (13, 18, 21, X and Y) accounted for only 25% of total abnormal chromosomes [45]. High aneuploid rates in human blastocysts were also reported in a recent study with 15,169 samples, overall in patients of 42–45 years old [46].

More euploid embryos can develop to blastocysts than aneuploid embryos. Arrested embryos are more likely to have abnormal chromosomes than developing embryos. High proportions of human embryos were aneuploid and the aneuploid rate increased with advanced maternal age. Interestingly, no significant difference was found in the developmental potential of embryos between younger patients and older patients.

In terms of monosomy and trisomy, no significant differences were found in the chromosomal distribution between blastocysts and arrested embryos. More arrested embryos had multiple chromosomal abnormalities than blastocysts. Errors occurred randomly in chromosomes, and there was no obvious difference between blastocysts and arrested embryos.

Aneuploidy could lead to reduced implantation and high miscarriage rates, but little is known about its mechanisms. Embryos usually arrest at various developmental stages for diverse reasons, such as culture conditions, patients' age and ovarian stimulation protocols. It is not known whether aneuploidy can directly influence embryo development. More euploid embryos developed to blastocyst than aneuploid embryos. These observations suggest that aneuploidy can affect embryo development in an unknown way or that the poorly understood factors that spoil euploidy also affects embryo development, for instance, energy impairment.

It was also observed that not only more arrested embryos were aneuploid, but also more chromosomes had errors in the arrested embryos than in blastocysts. It seems as a generalized failure. Many studies have been conducted to reveal the mechanisms of aneuploid origination in embryos from patients of advanced maternal age. It has been reported that maternal aging can dramatically influence the meiotic spindle assembly process in mammals [47] leading to spindle disorganization and chromosome segregation errors, which in turn cause aneuploid formation. Furthermore, the deterioration of sister chromatid cohesion and failure of the spindle assembly checkpoint in the oocytes are also crucial reasons for aneuploid formation [48], which mean a generalized failure. An aneuploid formation involves failure in many steps, which strongly suggest energy impairment.

The central problem in chromosome replication is generating two high-fidelity DNA copies and distributing them precisely to compartments that become the daughter cells. As cells grow, the mass of protein and membrane increases to a critical point that triggers the initiation of replication. Two replisomes are associated in a 'factory' that moves to the cell centre during chromosomal elongation. As DNA strands are pulled to the centre, replicated sister chromosomes migrate toward opposite cell poles. Completion of DNA synthesis occurs as the DNA that is pulled into the factory reaches the terminus. At this point, chromosomes are tangled together (catenated), and all physical connections must be removed to allow final separation. When physical separation is complete, cell wall synthesis forms two daughter cells.

In eukaryotic replication, initiation steps are not as fully understood as they are in *E. coli*. Initiation occurs at ***ars*** sites, so-called because they are autonomously replicating sequences. Initiation is controlled by a group of proteins called ORC (origin replication complex). Typically, a chromosome has many ORC-binding sites, and bidirectional semi-discontinuous forks move out from several ***ars*** sites on each chromosome until they converge with other forks. Eukaryotic replication also occurs in 'factories', and most of the chromosome is replicated in a semiconservative and semi-discontinuous mode, as in *E. coli*. The eukaryotic replication fork behaves very similarly to that found in *E. coli*.

Because replication is semi-discontinuous, the sister chromosomes are replication isomers. As replication proceeds, positive supercoils build up in front of the fork, and the daughter chromosomes become entangled behind the fork. One segment of a eukaryotic chromosome that is different from prokaryotic chromosomes is the tip of the chromosome, the telomere, which is replicated by a special DNA-polymerase called telomerase, which is related to the reverse transcriptase of retroviruses [49]. Telomerase synthesizes a simple repeat sequence that is added on to every chromosome using an RNA template that is part of the enzyme. In most organisms, telomerase is not expressed after cell differentiation, and consequently the telomere sequences shorten with age, eventually causing cell senescence and death. Following DNA replication in eukaryotes, which occurs in a part of the growth cycle called the S phase, cells move through a mechanical cycle called mitosis to distribute the replicated chromosomes to each daughter cell [50].

Mitosis proceeds through four stages. The first is the prophase in which, after replication, each chromosome becomes condensed. Stage 2 is metaphase, where two changes occur: each pair of replicated chromosomes moves to the cell centre and then the nuclear membrane begins to dissolve. In stage 3, anaphase, one centromere of each pair of chromosomes is attached to a set of fibers called the spindle, and molecular motors pull one of each chromosome pair to opposite cell poles. In stage 4, telophase, the nuclear membrane is reformed, and daughter cells are separated by the synthesis of a new septum [51].

The above brief description of a highly complex and accurate but at the same time poorly understood processes that lack a description about the role of energy generation and distribution, as it is usual in textbooks and research articles.

The organisms can adapt to widely varying growth states, from aerobic growth on rich nutrients to anaerobic growth in minimal salts and a single carbon and nitrogen source. One key to efficient growth is control of gene expression at the level of RNA transcription. The process of making of an RNA complement to a DNA gene is called transcription. The replication and transcription processes are not exempt from the use of energy in every one of its stages.

Because transcription and replication occur simultaneously, two situations arise where transcription machinery and replication machinery collide.

In eukaryotic chromosomes, the RNA polymerase responsible for transcribing most genes is remarkably similar at the structural level to the *E. coli* RNA polymerase. However, regulatory mechanisms are different. Eukaryotic genes have a region called the promoter which is where RNA polymerase binds and starts transcription. However, polymerase binding and its ability to initiate transcription is influenced by sites called transcription enhancers that can be upstream or downstream of the promoter (relative to the direction of transcription). Enhancers act over very large distances, and so DNA looping is required to bring enhancers into contact with RNA polymerase at promoters. In addition to enhancers, there are proteins called co-activators that must bind to RNA polymerase to stimulate transcription.

It is fascinating how mechanisms related to transcription and replication are described, but as usual, the role of energy is not mentioned at all.

Recombination is a critical repair pathway in mammalian chromosomes as well. Proteins that carry out biochemical reactions like the *E. coli* RecABC system have been identified. A protein called p53 coordinates the activity of many DNA repair proteins. Repair enzymes are stored at chromosome telomeres, and after a signal from p53, these proteins migrate to sites of DNA damage to restore chromosome function. Mutations in DNA repair genes have discovered to be responsible for several human genetic syndromes that result in premature ageing and high spontaneous rates of cancer. It is interesting how this highly complex machinery has been studied and patiently arranged; however, the role of generation and distribution of energy is fully relegated.

In eukaryotes, transposons (usually called retrotransposons because of their similarity to retroviruses and their dependence on reverse transcriptase for replication) make up a large fraction of total chromosomal DNA. In human cells, sequences called short interspersed nuclear elements (SINEs), which are about 300 bp long are present in about 106 copies and represent 5% of the mass of DNA in a haploid genome. One SINE, called AluI, is present on average once every 5000 bp in every human chromosome. There are also long interspersed nuclear elements (LINEs) of about 6 kb that are present in about 105 copies and represent 15% of the haploid chromosomal mass. What function, if any, these sequences provide for the host organism is questionable, but many genetic mutations have been attributed to gene disruption caused by recent transposon insertion. Cell uses energy in many ways, for instance in the careful arrangement of 6 kb, 5000 or 300 bp; besides to keep the form and to carry on their astonishing accurate function.

The published studies on this subject, despite how detailed they are, do not analyze two variables: energy levels and the presence of toxic molecules such as pesticides, herbicides, fertilizers, metals, plastics, solvents, industrial waste, anesthetic agents, etc.

Since embryological development to adulthood, melanin is so important, that it is present in every stage from the oocyte [52] to the mature adult organism.

7. Creatine kinase and ATP

Creatine kinase (CK), also known as creatine phosphokinase (COK) or phosphocreatine kinase, is an enzyme expressed by various tissues and cell types. CK catalyzes the conversion of creatine and uses adenosine triphosphate (ATP) to generate phosphocreatine (PCr) and adenosine diphosphate (ADP). This CK enzyme reaction is reversible and thus ATP can be generated from PCr and ADP.

Creatine kinase in the blood may be high in health and disease, for instance, exercise increases the outflow of creatine kinase to the blood stream for up to a week. Serum creatine kinase (CK) levels are reported to be around 70% higher in healthy black people, as compared with white people (median value 88 IU/L in white versus 149 IU/L in black people). Serum CK in healthy people is thought to occur from a proportional leak from normal tissues [53]. Creatine kinase (CK) activity in serum is widely used to diagnose tissue damage including myocardial infarction and skeletal muscle myopathy, but it is unknown why serum CK activity is higher in apparently healthy black people of sub-Saharan African descent [54], perhaps because more melanin means more available energy to impel both synthesis and function of creatine kinase.

There is no evidence of muscle damage in black people as cause for the high serum CK activity, and the BB, MB and MM isoenzymes in serum are proportionally higher, but have a normal distribution [55]. Serum CK in healthy subjects is supposedly to be derived from normal tissue "leaking" CK to lymphatic vessels and into the blood stream, proportionate to the intracellular CK concentration. Therefore, it was proposed that the black population subgroup has a generalized high CK activity in tissues, which means more energy expenditure.

CK activity in different types of tissues with high and fluctuating energy demands is higher in black people than in white people, independent of age. Normal tissue loses a small fraction of cytosolic CK into the interstitial space, as was shown in ^{31}P nuclear magnetic resonance spectroscopy studies [56]. In physiological and pathological states, release from tissue is proportional to tissue CK activity. Interstitial CK is subsequently transported through lymphatic vessels into the blood stream.

The unexplained high serum CK in healthy black people, with a normal isoenzyme distribution might be associated with a generalized high CK activity in tissues of this population subgroup. CK is the central regulatory enzyme of energy metabolism. The enzyme catalyzes the reversible transfer of the phosphoryl group (P) between creatine and ADP. CK supposedly fuels highly energy demanding processes such as cardiovascular contractility, sodium pumping and trophic responses, at a faster rate than glycolysis and oxidative phosphorylation together [57], however, the source of energy to CK system is poorly understood.

8. Glucose and ATP are not source of energy

The current dogma is that glucose is the universal precursor of any organic matter in plants and animals, human included. Glucose only provides highly specific carbon chains with which our body can synthesize and thereby replenishes organic molecules that wear out over the course of the day. The shape of carbon chains, of what we call glucose, seems to be very specific to the astonishing accurate metabolic processes of the human body and in general of all living beings, as they all contain glucose in their body. Glucose is arguably the ideal substrate or at least main substrate that fits appropriately into the sequence of highly complex and very specific metabolic processes of living beings. Thereby glucose is the universal provider of biomass, but no energy. If glucose were source of energy, diabetic patients should fly.

On the other hand, the ATP considered (wrongly) as the universal currency of energy exchange; it is a theory with significant contradictions. Although the theory was proposed more than 60 years ago, by Mitchell [58], who never worked on mitochondria, only on bacteria; in his chemiosmotic theory tried to establish the metabolic pathways about bioenergetics, which describes (theoretically) how living organisms acquire and transform energy in order to perform biological work. ATP is supposedly formed from adenosine diphosphate and inorganic phosphate. The overall reaction is catalyzed by ATP synthase, an enzyme that creates the energy storage molecule adenosine triphosphate (ATP), which is opposed to the law of thermodynamic that said that energy cannot be stored.

Mechanisms responsible for communication between spatially separated intracellular ATP consumption and ATP production process, and their precise coupling over a broad range of cellular functional activity has remained a longstanding enigma [59]. Optimal operation of the cellular bioenergetic system requires that energy-rich phosphoryl are produced and delivered to energy-consuming sites at the rate corresponding to the ATPase velocity, and that products of ATP hydrolysis, namely ADP, Pi and H^+, are removed in order to avoid kinetic and thermodynamic hindrances [60].

Cytoplasmic streaming, positioning of mitochondria and their movement in response to changes in energy utilization, along with formation of enzymatic complexes, have all been shown to contribute towards facilitating intracellular energetic communication [61]. However, such topological arrangements apparently are insufficient on their own to fulfill all cellular energetic needs [62]. Thereafter, a new theory of spatially arranged intracellular enzymatic networks, catalyzed by creatine kinase, adenylate kinase, carbonic anhydrase and glycolytic enzymes, in supporting high-energy phosphoryl transfer and signal communication between ATP-generating and ATP-consuming/ATP-sensing processes has implemented [63].

Fritz Lipman, the author of the energy concept through adenylate wire concept, was among the first to notice the analogy between the energy-carrying adenine nucleotide system and the electrical circuit. Indeed, basic principles of energy transfer, in terms of the rate and efficiency, apply equally to both industrial and metabolic networks [64]. In nature, the amount of energy tends to be constant in any system.

The localization of mitochondria in close proximity to cellular energy-utilizing processes, and their movement in response to activation of ATP-utilizing reactions [65], suggest that the distance of energy transfer is critical for adequate energy supply. It is hard to accept that mitochondria are in close proximity to cellular energy-utilizing processes, for instance, cell nucleus has neither mitochondria nor ATP, in spite to be the largest organelle with a high energy consumption; furthermore, energy transfer by diffusional exchange of adenine nucleotides is kinetically and thermodynamically inefficient since it requires a significant concentration gradient [66] and would result in ATPase inhibition by end products (Pi, ADP and H^+), inability to sustain the high free energy of ATP hydrolysis (ΔGATP) at sites of ATP utilization, and ultimately energy dissipation (–ΔH) during transmission [67]. The difference between ΔG1(ATP) and ΔG2(ATP), signifying energy loss (–ΔH), would increase at higher rates of ATP turnover, and the drop of ΔG2(ATP) below a threshold would impair cellular functions [68].

Part of intracellular energy transfer proceeds in the narrow mitochondrial inner membrane infoldings, known as cristae. The cristae arrangement increases, by several folds, the capacity of mitochondrial ATP production without occupying additional intracellular space. However, it creates difficulties in ATP export from the mitochondrial intra-cristae space, as diffusional flux requires a significant concentration gradient. Accordingly, ATP accumulation in the mitochondrial intra-cristae space would inhibit export of ATP from the mitochondrial matrix by locking the adenine nucleotide translocator [69].

The disruption of the adenylate kinase gene impedes ATP export from mitochondria [70]. Taken together, this would indicate that in the absence of facilitating mechanisms, cell architecture and diffusional hindrances would obstruct free movement of molecules, impeding efficient intracellular communication.

In searching how cells overcome diffusional limitations for substrate development [71] several theories have been implemented. However, is difficult to explain the displacement of the local ATP/ADP equilibrium to other cellular sites to maintain energetic homeostasis [72]. Understanding of creatine kinase function was specially limited when the cell is considered as a homogenous system where enzymes are in equilibrium, and metabolites have uniform distributions and concentrations [73], without forgetting the energy, which also remains constant.

Past observations following deletion of brain B-CK indicate that this isoform is fundamental to processes that involve habituation, spatial learning and seizure susceptibility [74]; however, these effects can be explained by the effect on thermoregulation of mitochondria and CK, more than an energy source effect. The reduction in cellular B-CK activity by dominant negative gene expression abrogates thrombin-mediated, energy-dependent signal transduction during cytoskeletal reorganization [75]; which are varied effects that are difficult to explain from a purely biochemical point of view, except if we take into account the fundamental role of energy.

The muscle exercise performance correlates with adenylate kinase activity, suggesting that this enzyme is an integral part of cellular energetic homeostasis [76], but explainable by its effect on thermic regulation that is astonishingly accurate; more than some effect on generation and distribution of energy from melanin.

It is possible that the main function of mitochondria and ATP is temperature control, as intracellular chemical reactions require (constantly) not only the exact reactants, the exact energy, but also the exact temperature (**Figure 4**).

ATP is thermodynamically unstable and electrochemically stable. When ATP is hydrolyzed to ADP energy is absorbed, and when the ADP is scaled to ATP the energy is released. The characteristics of these reactions are compatible with temperature regulation, as they happen quickly and constantly, as each ATP molecule in the body requires reconstitution every 20 s.

It is pertinent to emphasize that ATP hydrolysis and reconstitution also requires, like any other chemical process of the body or cell, energy at each and every stage of the reaction. The unsuspected intrinsic property of melanin to transform sunlight into chemical energy by dissociating the molecule from water, such as chlorophyll in plants; allows to rethink cell biology in a new way completely different, and chromosomes are not exception.

Thereby, the precise coupling of spatially separated intracellular ATP-producing and ATP-consuming processes is a formidable challenge, and even more so in an organelle that lacks mitochondria and ATP as is the nucleus of the eukaryotic cell.

The role of adenine nucleotides as a supposedly key link between spatially separated energy transducing processes, still it is a theory after almost 80 years that was proposed by Lipmann in 1941. The adenylate wire theory has many contradictions, such as the distance of energy transfer is critical for adequate energy supply, it requires a significant concentration gradient, could be ATPase inhibition by end products; the ΔG_{ATP} is difficult to maintain in the adequate levels at sites of ATP utilization; and finally energy dissipation ($-\Delta H$) during transmission.

The difference between $\Delta G_{1(ATP)}$ and $\Delta G_{2(ATP)}$, signifying energy loss ($-\Delta H$), would increase at higher rates of ATP turnover, and the drop of $\Delta G_{2(ATP)}$ below a threshold would impair cellular functions [68]. Therefore, energy management is very complicated and difficult to explain and understand whether we start from glucose and ATP as an energy source. But if we divide from now on the energy (light/melanin/water) of the mass (glucose), things will change for the sake of the health of the sick.

Supposedly, part of intracellular energy transfer proceeds in the narrow mitochondrial inner membrane infoldings, known as cristae. The cristae arrangement increases, by several folds, the capacity of mitochondrial ATP production without occupying additional intracellular space. However, it creates difficulties in ATP export from the mitochondrial intracristae space, as diffusional flux requires a significant concentration gradient. Therefore, ATP accumulation in the mitochondrial intracristae space would inhibit export of ATP from the mitochondrial matrix by locking the adenine nucleotide translocator [77]. It is very difficult just to explain

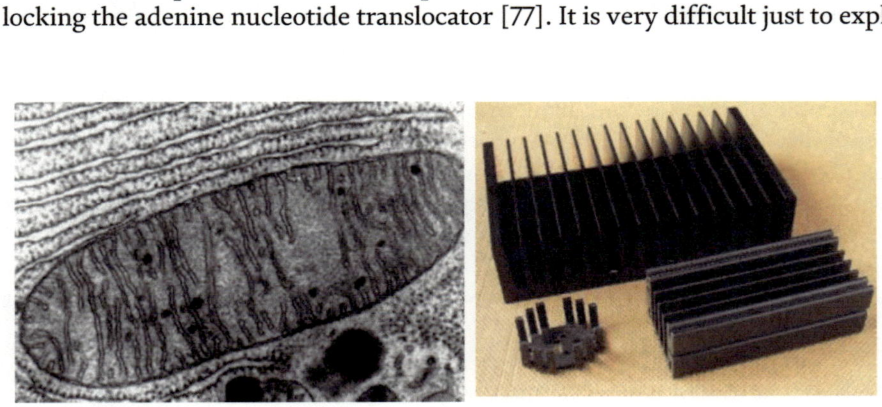

Figure 4.
The morphology of mitochondria (left) is similar to heat sinks (right) used in electronic devices and some light sources.

the generation and distribution of energy from glucose and ATP. And just as you cannot take more energy than a molecule or system has, it is also not possible to explain the inexplicable because it's simply not possible.

The normal cell architecture and the diffusional hindrances seems to be designated to obstruct free movement of molecules, impeding efficient intracellular communication, the generation and distribution of energy from glucose and/or ATP. On the one hand, if energy management were so difficult, life would be a miracle and not an evolution, and on the other hand, if glucose were a source of energy, diabetics would fly.

The field of how cells overcome diffusional limitations for substrate movement in the highly structured intracellular milieu is full of theories. Concepts as displacement of equilibrium, near-equilibrium network, sharp concentration waveform, incoming flux wave, flux transfers chains, instantaneous transmission, vectorial ligand conduction, chains of sequential rapid equilibrating reactions, facilitated high-energy phosphoryl transfer are theories initially developed by Peter Mitchel and have gradually been added by other researchers with biochemical "patches" trying to make them believable [78]. But it is not possible to extract energy from where there is none.

Interestingly, there is theory named "walking without moving" that means that ligands do not move the entire length of the pathway, as molecules arriving at the distal sites of this sequence represent the equivalent rather than the specific molecule generated at the origination site [79]; explanation is not simple and more than complex tangled mechanisms are being argued. For instance, it is said that flux wave propagation along rapid equilibrating chemical and biological reaction can proceed much faster than diffusion of reactants [80], but only gases move faster in aqueous solution than the electrolytes contained in it.

And now that we know that melanin releases molecular hydrogen and molecular oxygen continuously, we will have to include these gases in the schemes of intracellular biochemical reactions.

The purpose of this work is not the exhaustive analysis of all the contradictions of the intracellular biochemical pathways described to date in the literature, we only explain some demonstrative examples of the excessive complexity that has been reached trying to explain the prevailing theories and dogmas.

9. Light transduction by melanin and chlorophyll

Photosynthesis, a major bioenergetic process, is the metabolic pathway used by plants in which solar energy is used to synthesize glucose from carbon dioxide and water. This reaction takes place in the chloroplast. After glucose is synthesized, the plant cell can undergo photophosphorylation to produce ATP [81]. To date, it was not known that humans or mammals in general could carry out a transduction of luminous energy to chemical energy from dissociation of water, such as plants (**Figure 5**). However, the study of the minuscule vessels of the optic nerve in humans (**Figure 6**) and their reaction to the presence of melanin came to reveal the unsuspected intricate property of melanin to dissociate and reform the molecule of water [82].

The task ahead is to integrate the unsuspected bioenergy role of melanin into today's biochemical tangle. It is to be hoped that the requirement of philosophers that science has to be simple will be fulfilled. To the definition of life as a self-sustaining chemical system that eventually enters into Darwinian development, we can now add: life is a self-sustaining physical-chemical system capable of evolving.

Chlorophyll:

$$2H_2O \longrightarrow 2H_2 + O_2$$

Melanin:

$$2H_2O \longrightarrow 2H_2 + O_2 \longrightarrow 2H_2O + 4e^-$$

Figure 5.
Water dissociation is irreversible in chlorophyll; however, in melanin it is reversible.

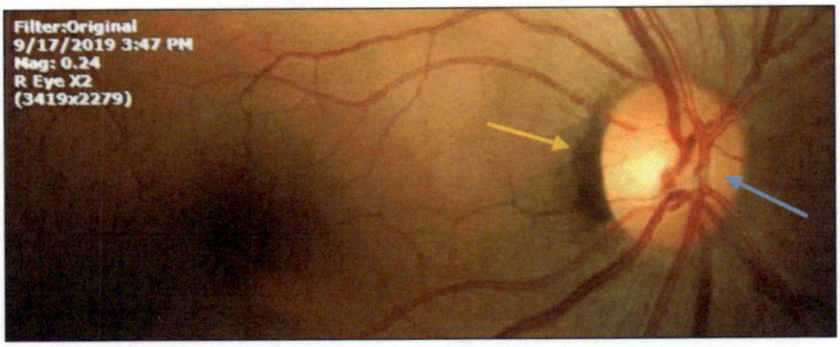

Figure 6.
The optic nerve (blue arrow) and melanin (yellow arrow) are always together with a very interesting crosstalk.

10. Conclusion

In biology, nothing makes sense except in the light of evolution. The origin of life could not be explained from glucose, genes or chromosomes. Nor has it been able to be explained from the ATP. But it is that ATP is not a source of energy, the functions of ATP are different, and you will have to discern them, perhaps it is for temperature control and control of inorganic phosphorus levels.

Therefore, the origin of life could not be explained from the energy of the ATP either. But things change when we understand the unsuspected bioenergy role of melanin in biology. Melanin is the most stable substance known, 160 million years of age. A source of energy so stable and accurate at the same time, allows to order the ideas as to the origin of life, because then we would have, at the beginning of time: melanin, the energy emanating from melanin, then glucose, then more complex molecules such as amino acids, lipids, nucleic acids, etc.

Then the order of the origin of life would look like this: melanin, melanin energy, glucose, amino acids, lipids, proteins (histones), nucleic acids (genes) and so on. Therefore, before the genes was melanin and the energy that comes from it.

Usually, when we talk about genetic alterations, we usually think that before the genes there is nothing, evolutionarily speaking, but now we must be aware that, before the genes is the origin of life, which is explained by the melanin and the energy that emanates of her.

Therefore, chromosomal abnormalities at the chromosome level, at the gene level, at the order level of nucleic acids or even histones can be explained by alterations in the generation and distribution of energy that comes from melanin, which does not glucose or ATP.

In any system, when failure is widespread, we must first think about energy. And in the case of chromosomal abnormalities the alterations are diffuse, are not punctual or limited to a single gene or even a single chromosome. And even alterations extended to anatomical malformations, which is consistent with widespread failure; and now that we know that the main energy source of the cell, tissues, organs, systems or the human body as a whole comes from melanin, then the alterations observed at the various levels of organization, correspond to a generalized failure, typical alterations in energy generation and distribution.

Our discovery about the intrinsic property of melanin to dissociate the molecule from water is a disruptive finding that breaks into a thousand pieces the sacrosanct role of glucose as an energy source and at the same time opens new paths that will allow us to advance in knowledge of the intricate mysteries of life.

We must rewrite cell biology completely, re-thinking organelle functions based on the discovery that eukaryote cells are able to directly take energy from light. In this chapter, we will give some examples of how the relevant role of energy in the cell nucleus and in the dynamic of chromosomes has been systematically relegated in the study of the biology of chromosomes.

Explaining something completely different from established dogmas is not simple, it is necessary to explain step by step the interpretation errors of glucose-based metabolism as an energy source; there are concepts that the reader will have to unlearn and implement other constructs not only with what he will read here, but in other sources of information, so that he structures a totally different picture from what is known. We aspire to be a first approach with a discovery that will mark a before and after in the study, in the case of this chapter; of the chromosomal abnormalities.

Acknowledgements

This work was supported by Human Photosynthesis® Research Centre, Aguascalientes 20000, México.

Author details

Arturo Solis Herrera
Human Photosynthesis® Research Centre, Aguascalientes, Mexico

*Address all correspondence to: comagua2000@yahoo.com

References

[1] Available from: www.ggu.ac.in [Retrieved: 4 November 2019]

[2] Available from: www.biology.ke nyon.edu [Retrieved: 4 November 2019]

[3] Gardner RJM. Chromosomes and clinical anatomy. Clinical Anatomy. 2016;**29**(5):540-546

[4] Higgings NP. Introductory article. Encyclopedia of Life Sciences. Macmillan Publishers LTD. Nature Publishers Group; 2001. Available from: ///G:/Documents/Documents/Arturo%20Solìs%20Herrera/Artículos%20en%20progreso/Intech%20Oct%2010%202018%20Chapter/2019%20Chromosomic%20abnormalities/cromosomeStructure.pdf [Retrieved: 14 August 1019]

[5] Gibcus HS, Dekker J. The hierarchy of the 3D genome. Molecular Cell. 2013; **49**:773-782. DOI: 10.1016/j.molcell.2013.02.011

[6] Finn EH, Misteli T. Molecular basis and biological function of variability in spatial genome organization. Science. 2019;**365**(6457):eaaw9498. DOI: 10.1126/science.aaw9498

[7] Parada LA, Roix JJ, Misteli T. A uncertainity principle in chromosome positioning. Trends in Cell Biology. 2003;**13**:393-396. DOI: 10.1016/SO962-8924(03)00149-1

[8] Schoenfelder S et al. Preferential associations between co-regulated genes reveal a transcriptional interactome in erythroid cells. Nature Genetics. 2010; **42**:53-61. DOI: 10.1038/ng496

[9] Yunger SR, Garini L, Shav-Tai Y. Single-allele analysis of transcription kinetics in living mammalian cells. Nature Methods. 2010;7:631-633. DOI: 10.1038/nmeth.1482

[10] Lenstra TL, Rodriguez J, Chen H, Larson DR. Transcription dynamics in living cells. Annual Review of Biophysics. 2016;**45**:25-27. DOI: 10.1146/annurev-biophys-062215-010838

[11] Symmons O, Raj A. What´s luck go to do with it: Single cells, multiple fates, and biological non-determinism. Molecular Cell. 2016;**62**:788-802. DOI: 10.1016/j.molcell 2016.05.023

[12] Szabo Q et al. TADs are structural 3D units of high order chromosome organization in Drosophilia. Science Advances. 2018;**4**:Eear8082. DOI: 10.1126/sciadv.aar8082

[13] Finn EH et al. Extensive heterogeneity and intrinsic variation in Spatial Genome Organization. Cell. 2019;**176**:1502-1515e10

[14] Tiana G et al. Structural fluctuations of the chromatin fiber within topologically association domains. Biophysical Journal. 2016;**110**: 1234-1245. DOI: 101016/j.bpj2016.02.003

[15] Hansen AS, Pustova I, Cattoglio C, Tijan R, Darzacq X. CTCF and cohesin regulate chromatin loop stability with distinct dynamics. eLife. 2017;**6**:e25776. DOI: 10.7554/elife25776

[16] Cattoni DI et al. Single cell absolute contact probability detection reveals chromosomes are organized by multiple low frequencies yet specific interactions. Nature Communications. 2017;**8**:1753. DOI: 10.1038/s41467-017-01962-x

[17] Stevens TJ et al. 3D structures of individual mammalian genomes, studied by single cell H-C. Nature. 2017; **544**:59-64. DOI: 10.1038/nature21429

[18] Perkel JM. Chromatin untangled: New methods map genomic structure.

Science. 2016;**354**(6308):118-120. DOI: 10.1126/science.354.6308.118

[19] Kosak ST et al. Subnuclear compartmentalization of immunoglobulinloci during lymphocyte development. Science. 2002;**296**: 158-162. DOI: 101126/science1068768

[20] Lyons BD et al. Heterochromatin-mediated gene silencing facilitates the diversification of olfactory neurons. Cell Reports. 2014;**9**:884-982. DOI: 10.1016/celrep.2014.10.001

[21] Branciamore S et al. Frequent monoallelic or skewed expression for developmental genes in CNS-derived cells and evidence for balancing selection. Proceedings of the National Academy of Sciences of the United States of America. 2018;**115**:E10379-E10386. DOI: 10.1073/pnas.1808652115

[22] Tan L, Xing D, Chang C, Li H, Xie XS. Three-dimensional genome structures of single diploid human cells. Science. 2018;**361**:924-928. DOI: 10.1126/science.aa15641

[23] Chubb JR, Boyle S, Perry P, Bickmore WA. Chromatin motion is constrained by association with nuclear compartments in human cells. Current Biology. 2002;**12**:439-445. DOI: 101016/SO960-9822(02)00695-4

[24] Vivante A, Brozgol E, Bronshtein I, Gariny Y. Genome organization in the nucleus: From dynamic measurements to a functional model. Methods: A Companion to Methods in Enzymology. 2017;**123**:128-137. DOI: 10.1016/j.ymeth.2017.01.008

[25] Lim B, Heist T, Levine M, Fukaya T. Visualization of transvection in living Drosophilia embryos. Molecular Cell. 2018;**70**:287-296 e6. DOI: 101016/j.molcel2018.02.09

[26] Soutouglou E, Misteli T. On the contribution of spatial genome organization to cancerous chromosome translocations. Journal of the National Cancer Institute Monographs. 2008; **2008**:16-19. DOI: 10.1093/jncimonographs/Ign07

[27] Drubin DA, Garakani AM, Silver PA. Motion as phenotype: The use of live-cell imaging and machine visual screening to characterize transcription-dependent chromosome dynamics. BMC Cell Biology. 2006;**7**:19. DOI: 10.1186/1471-2121-7-19

[28] Sinha DK, Banerjee B, Maharana S, Shivashankar GV. Probing the dynamic organization of transcription compartments and gene loci within the nucleus of living cells. Biophysical Journal. 2008;**95**:5432-5438. DOI: 10.1529/byophysj.108135921

[29] Marshal AD et al. CTCF genetic alterations in endometrial carcinoma are pro-tumorigenic. Oncogene. 2017;**36**: 4100-4110. DOI: 10.1038/onc.2017.25

[30] Torres CM et al. The linker histone H1.0 generates epigenetic and functional intratumor heterogeneity. Science. 2016;**353**:Aaf1644. DOI: 10.1126/science.aaf1644

[31] Higgins NP. Chromosome structure. In: Encyclopedia of Life Sciences. Macmillan Publishers LTD, Nature Publishing Group; 2001. DOI: 10.1038/npg.els.0001486

[32] Dzeja PP, Bortolon R, Perez-Terzic C, Holmuhamedov EL, Terzic A. Energetic communication between mitochondria and nucleus directed by catalyzed phosphotransfer. Proceedings of the National Academy of Sciences of the United States of America. 2002;**99**: 10156-10161

[33] Kuzminov A. Recombinational repair of DNA damage in *Escherichia coli* and bacteriophage l. Microbiology and Molecular Biology Reviews. 1999;**63**: 751-813

[34] Casjens S. Bacterial genome structure. Annual Review of Genetics. 1998;**32**:339-377

[35] Bruces A, Johnson A. The global structure of chromosomes. In: Molecular Biology of the Cell. 4th ed. New York; 2002 Garland Science

[36] Alberts B, Johnson A, Lewis J, et al. DNA and chromosomes. In: Alberts B, Johnson A, Lewis J, et al., editors. Molecular Biology of the Cell. 4th ed. New York: Garland Science; 2002

[37] Dame RT. The role of nucleoid-associated proteins in the organization and compaction of bacterial chromatin. Molecular Microbiology. 2005;**56**(4): 858-870. DOI: 10.1111/ j.1365-2958.2005.04598.x

[38] Allemand JF, Bensimon D, Croquette V. Strechting DNA and RNA to probe their interactions with proteins. Current Opinion in Structural Biology. 2003;**13**:266-10663

[39] Gorin MB. When Genetics Can Point Researchers and clinicians in new directions. JAMA Ophthalmology. 2019; **137**(8):876-877. DOI: 10.1001/ jamaophthalmol.2019.1325

[40] Berger SI, Iyengar R. Network analyses in systems pharmacology. Bioinformatics. 2009;**25**(19):2466-2472. DOI: 10.1093/bioinformatics/btp465

[41] Gorin MB, Weeks DE, Baron RV, Conley YP, Ortube MC, Nusinowitz S. Endophenotypes for age-related macular degeneration: Extending our reach into the preclinical stages of disease. Journal of Clinical Medicine. 2014;**3**(4):1335-1356. DOI: 10.3390/ jcm3041335

[42] Pauling L, Itano HA, Singer SJ, Wells IC. Sickle cell anemia, a molecular disease. Science. 1949;**110**:543-547

[43] Velde ER, Pearson PL. The variability of female reproductive ageing. Human Reproduction Update. 2002;**8**:141-154

[44] Qi ST, Xian X, Liu J-Q, Wang W. Arrested human embryos are more likely to have abnormal chromosomes than developing embryos from women of advanced maternal age. Journal of Ovarian Research. 2014;**7**:65

[45] Baart EB, Martini E, Van den Berg I, Macklon NS, Galjaard RJ. Preimplantation genetic screening reveals a high incidence of aneuploidy and mosaicism in embryos from young women undergoing IVF. Human Reproduction. 2006;**21**:223-233

[46] Franasiak JM, Forman EJ, Hong KH, Werner MD, Upham KM. The nature of aneuploidy with increasing age of female partner: A review of 15,169 consecutive trophectoderm biopsies evaluated with comprehensive chromosomal screening. Fertility and Sterility. 2014;**101**:656-663

[47] Battaglia DE, Goodwin P, Klein NA, Soules MR. Influence of maternal age on meiotic spindle assembly in oocytes from naturally cycling women. Human Reproduction. 1996;**1**:2217-2222

[48] Wang ZB, Chatten H, Sun QY. Why chromosome segregation error in oocytes increased with maternal aging? Physiology (Bethesda). 2011;**26**:314-325

[49] Esposito D, Petrovic A, Harris R, Ono S, et al. H-NS oligomerization domain structure reveals the mechanism for high order self-association of the intact protein. Journal of Molecular Biology. 2002;**324**:841-450

[50] Skoko D, Wong B, Johnson RC, Marko JF. Micromechanical analysis of the binding of DNA-bending proteins HMGB1, NHP6A, and HU reveals their ability to form highly stable DNA-proteins complexes. Biochemistry. 2004;**43**:13867-13874

[51] Zhang J, Zeuner Y, Kleefeld A, Unden G, Janshoff A. Multiple site-specific binding of Fis protein to *Escherichia coli* nuoA-N promoter DNA and its impact onDNA topology visualised by means of scanning forcemicroscopy. Chembiochem. 2004; **5**:1286

[52] Harsa-King M. Melanogenesis in oocytes of wild type and mutant albino axolotls. Developmental Biology. 1980; **74**:251-262

[53] Brewster LM, Coronel CMD, Sluiter W, Clark JF, van Montfrans GA. Ethnic differences in tissue creatine kinase activity: An observational study. PLoS One. 2012;**7**(3):e32471. Available from: https://doi.org/10.1371/journal.pone.0032471

[54] Brewster LM, Mairuhu G, Sturk A, van Montfrans GA. Distribution of creatine kinase in the general population: Implications for statin therapy. American Heart Journal. 2007; **154**:655-661

[55] Apple FS, Quist HE, Doyle PJ, Otto AP, Murakami MM. Plasma 99th percentile reference limits for cardiac troponin and creatine kinase MB mass for use with European Society of Cardiology/American College of Cardiology consensus recommendations. Clinical Chemistry. 2003;**49**:1331-1336

[56] West-Jordan JA, Martin PA, Abraham RJ, Edwards RH, Jackson MJ. Energy dependence of cytosolic enzyme efflux from rat skeletal muscle. Clinica Chimica Acta. 1990;**189**:163-172

[57] Djeza PP, Terzic A. Phosphotransfer networks and cellular energetics. The Journal of Experimental Biology. 2003; **206**:2039-2047

[58] Mitchell P. Coupling of phosphorylation to electron and hydrogen transfer by a chemi-osmotic type of mechanism. Nature. 1961; **191**(4784):144-148. PMID: 13771349. DOI: 10.1038/191144a0

[59] Ames A III. CNS energy metabolism as related to function. Brain Research. Brain Research Reviews. 2000;**34**:42-68

[60] Dzeja PP, Redfield MM, Burnett JC, Terzic A. Failing energetics in failing hearts. Current Cardiology Reports. 2000;**2**:212-217

[61] Lange S, Auerbach D, McLoughlin P, Perriard E, Schafer BW, Perriard JC, et al. Subcellular targeting of metabolic enzymes to titin in heart muscle may be mediated by DRAL/FHL-2. Journal of Cell Science. 2002;**115**: 4925-4936

[62] de Groof AJ, Oerlemans FT, Jost CR, Wieringa B. Changes in glycolytic network and mitochondrial design in creatine kinase-deficient muscles. Muscle & Nerve. 2001;**24**:1188-1196

[63] Joubert F, Mazet JL, Mateo P, Hoerter JA. 31P NMR detection of subcellular creatine kinase fluxes in the perfused rat heart: Contractility modifies energy transfer pathways. The Journal of Biological Chemistry. 2002; **277**:1846918476

[64] Jeong H, Tombor B, Albert R, Oltvai ZN, Barabasi AL. The large-scale organization of metabolic networks. Nature. 2000;**407**:651-654

[65] Hollenbeck PJ. The pattern and mechanism of mitochondrial transport in axons. Frontiers in Bioscience. 1996;**1**: D91-D102

[66] Jacobus WE. Respiratory control and the integration of heart high energy phosphate metabolism by mitochondrial creatine kinase. Annual Review of Physiology. 1985;**47**:707-725

[67] Kammermeier H. Myocardial cell energetics. Advances in Experimental Biology. 1997;**430**:89-96

[68] Taegtmeyer H. Genetics of energetics: Transcriptional responses in cardiac metabolism. Annals of Biomedical Engineering. 2000;**28**: 871-876

[69] Mannella CA, Pfeiffer DR, Bradshaw PC, Moraru II, Slepchenko B, Loew LM, et al. Topology of the mitochondrial inner membrane: Dynamics and bioenergetic implications. IUBMB Life. 2001;**52**: 93-100

[70] Bandlow W, Strobel G, Zoglowek C, Oechsner U, Magdolen V. Yeast adenylate kinase is active simultaneously in mitochondria and cytoplasm and is required for non-fermentative growth. European Journal of Biochemistry. 1988;**178**:451-457

[71] Nagle S. Regulation problems in the energy metabolism of the myocardium (germ). Klinische Wochenschrift. 1970; **48**:1075-1089

[72] Dzeja PP, Terzic A, Wieringa B. Phosphotransfer dynamics in skeletal muscle from creatine kinase gene-deleted mice. Molecular and Cellular Biochemistry. 2004;**256-257**(1-2):13-27. PMID: 14977167. DOI: 10.1023/b:mcbi.0000009856.23646.38

[73] Kushmerick MJ. Skeletal muscle: A paradigm for testing principles of bioenergetics. Journal of Bioenergetics and Biomembranes. 1995;**27**:555-569

[74] Jost CR, Van Der Zee CE, In't Zandt HJ, Oerlemans F, Verheij M, Streijger F, et al. Creatine kinase B-driven energy transfer in the brain is important for habituation and spatial learning behaviour, mossy fibre field size and determination of seizure susceptibility. The European Journal of Neuroscience. 2002;**15**:1692-1706

[75] Mahajan VB, Pai KS, Lau A, Cunningham DD. Creatine kinase, an ATP-generating enzyme, is required for thrombin receptor signaling to the cytoskeleton. Proceedings of the National Academy of Sciences of the United States of America. 2000;**97**: 12062-12067

[76] Linossier MT, Dormois D, Fouquet R, Geyssant A, Denis C. Use of the forcevelocity test to determine the optimal braking force for a sprint exercise on a friction-loaded cycle ergometer. European Journal of Applied Physiology and Occupational Physiology. 1996;**74**:420-427

[77] Slepchenko B, Loew LM, Hsieh CE, Buttle K, Marko M. Topology of the mitochondrial inner membrane: Dynamics and bioenergetic implications. IUBMB Life. 2001;**52**: 93-100

[78] Mitchell P. Compartmentation and communication in living systems. Ligand conduction: A general catalytic principle in chemical, osmotic and chemiosmotic reaction systems. European Journal of Biochemistry. 1979; **95**:1-20

[79] Tuckerman ME, Marx D, Parrinello M. The nature and transport mechanism of hydrated hydroxide ions in aqueous solution. Nature. 2002;**417**: 925-929

[80] Mair T, Muller SC. Traveling NADH and proton waves during oscillatory glycolysis in vitro. The Journal of Biological Chemistry. 1996;**271**:627-630

[81] Nelson DL, Cox MM. Lehninger: Principles of Biochemistry. 6th ed. New York: W.H. Freeman and Company; 2013. p. 731

[82] Herrera AS, Esparza MC, Ghulam A, Zamyatnin AA Jr, Aliev G. Beyond mitochondria, what would be the energy source of the cell? Central Nervous System Agents in Medicinal Chemistry. 2015;**15**:32-41

Section 3

Chromosomal Abnomalities Observed in Plants

Chapter 8

Polyploidy in the Ginger Family from Thailand

Kesara Anamthawat-Jónsson and Puangpaka Umpunjun

Abstract

Polyploidy is common in the ginger family Zingiberaceae. The aims of the present paper are (1) to provide a general introduction on species diversity with emphasis on conservation; (2) to highlight the human-use significance of this family, focusing on the two major genera, *Zingiber* (ginger) and *Curcuma* (turmeric); (3) to present chromosome number data from 45 natural and cultivated *Curcuma* taxa from Thailand, of which polyploids are predominant; and (4) to describe our own work on cytotaxonomy of selected Thai *Curcuma* species. We obtained somatic chromosome numbers from root tips and analysed meiotic chromosome behaviour from flowers. We also used the molecular cytogenetic method of ribosomal gene mapping on chromosomes to infer mechanism of polyploidization and reveal genomic relationships among closely related species. The main results of our cytogenetic studies include the following. The most sought-after medicinal *Curcuma* cultivars growing on a large-scale basis are secondary triploids, so as taxa in natural habitats that are harvested for local utilisation. These triploids are sexually deficient, due to meiotic pairing abnormalities, but they are propagated asexually via rhizomes. The ribosomal mapping results indicate natural triploidization process via hybridisation, either within populations or across the species boundaries.

Keywords: *Curcuma*, cytogenetics, cytotaxonomy, ethnobotany, ginger, medicinal plants, polyploidy, triploidy, turmeric, *Zingiber*

1. Introduction

Taxonomic classification of the ginger family (Zingiberaceae) is still under revision for many floras, as more than 3000 species names have been used worldwide, but only half of these are accepted. These aromatic herbs grow in moist areas of the tropics and subtropics, including some regions that are seasonably dry. The ginger family comprises about 50 genera and more than 1300 species worldwide, and in Thailand 21 genera with about 200 species have been described. Numerous species are endemic to Thailand, but the majority has a wider distribution, especially over Southeast and South Asia. A few species of this family are commercially cultivated, such as ginger (*Zingiber officinale* Rosc.), turmeric (*Curcuma longa* L.) and aromatic ginger (*Kaempferia galanga* L.). Interestingly, these widely cultivated species are sexually deficient triploid or pentaploid plants—the elite cultivars are therefore propagated by rhizomes. These polyploid species are superior to their diploid relatives in terms of growth and yield, while the sought-after quality characters remain unchanged.

2. The ginger family (Zingiberaceae), with emphasis on *Curcuma*

The ginger family or Zingiberaceae comprises about 50 genera and more than 1300 species worldwide [1, 2]. The family distribution is pantropical, with centre of species diversity in South and Southeast Asia. Some species are found in America and subtropical and warm-temperate Asia. In China, 20 genera and 216 species (141 endemic, four introduced) have been recorded [1]. Geographically, Thailand is part of the Indochinese region that harbours the highest ginger genetic resources [3, 4]. Several of these species are rare and endemic to Thailand [5]. A large number of Thai taxa of Zingiberaceae are known as edible, ornamental or medicinal plants, from which commercial products beneficial to human can be developed.

Two best known genera in the context of cultivation and human uses worldwide are *Zingiber* Miller (ginger) and *Curcuma* Linnaeus (turmeric). The largest genus *Zingiber*, which comprises 100–200 species, is native to Southeast Asia especially in Thailand [6], China [7], the Indian subcontinent and New Guinea [8]. It contains the true gingers, plants grown for their medicinal and culinary value. The best known is *Z. officinale*, the garden ginger.

Curcuma is a genus of about 120 accepted species in the family Zingiberaceae that contains such species as turmeric (*C. longa*) and Siam tulip (*C. alismatifolia* Gagnep.). They are native to Southeast Asia, southern China, the Indian subcontinent, New Guinea and northern Australia [6, 8–11]. Tropical Asia and South Asia are the diversity hotspots of the genus. Although the species diversity is very high and new species are being discovered regularly, other species are disappearing. Habitat loss, due to global warming, deforestation, agricultural expansion and anthropogenic activities, is one of the main causes of biodiversity loss worldwide [12–14]. In addition, overharvesting for use in traditional medicine has raised a serious concern that wild plants will be disappearing from nature.

According to the IUCN Red List of Threatened Species, seven *Curcuma* species have been declared endangered to extinction (EN) and six additionally critically endangered (CR). The endemic EN species are *C. caulina* J. Graham, India [15]; *C. colorata* Valeton, Indonesia [16]; *C. coriacea* Mangaly & M. Sabu, India [17]; *C. corniculata* Skornick., Lao [18]; *C. prasina* Skornick., Thailand [19]; *C. sahuynhensis* Skornick. & N.S. Lý, Vietnam [20]; and *C. vitellina* Skornick. & H.D.Tran, Vietnam [21]. The endemic CR species are *C. bhatii* (R.M.Sm.) Skornick. & M. Sabu, India [22]; *C. leonidii* Skornick. & Luu, Vietnam [23]; *C. newmanii* Skornick., Vietnam [24]; *C. pygmaea* Skornick. & Sida f., Vietnam [25]; *C. supraneeana* (W.J. Kress & K. Larsen) Skornick., Thailand [26]; and *C. vamana* M. Sabu and Mangaly, India [27]. There clearly is an urgent need to protect these *Curcuma* species in their natural habitats while at the same time encouraging ex situ conservation and supporting researches aiming to find viable methods for sustainable cultivation of species of economic potential.

3. Recent publications on the ginger family

The survey of recent (2019) publications on Zingiberaceae in the Web-of-Science database, using "ginger" as keyword in titles (**Figure 1**), shows that the genus *Zingiber* (ginger) is by far the most investigated worldwide. The most researched topics concern medicinal properties and health benefits of ginger (1); pharmaceutical, biochemical and molecular characterisation (2); applications in food science and chemistry (3); other technologies and industrial applications (4); as well as some effort in improving cultivation (5). On the other hand, research on *Zingiber* diversity, taxonomy, ecology and genetics (6) is limited.

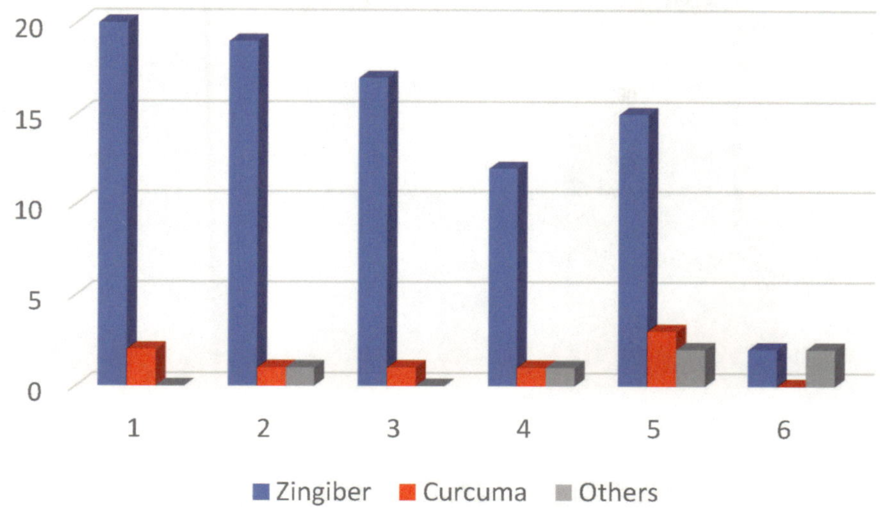

Figure 1.
Distribution of recent publications by research topics in 2019, obtained from web-of-science database (webofknowledge.com/WOS_), using the single keyword "ginger" in title. Research topics (x-axis): 1, medicinal properties and health benefits; 2, pharmaceutical, biochemical and molecular research; 3, food science and chemistry; 4, other technologies and industrial applications; 5, cultivation and agriculture; and 6, biodiversity, taxonomy, ecology and genetics. Y-axis: Percentages of the number of publications in 166 totals. Blue columns include papers on Zingiber, *ginger, gingerols and ginger-related topics. Red columns include papers on* Curcuma, *turmeric, curcumins and related topics. Grey columns include other species in the ginger family Zingiberaceae.*

Ginger (*Z. officinale*) is a very popular spice used worldwide, whether it be used to spice up meals, or as a medicine [28]. Ginger can be used for a variety of food or medicine items, as vegetables, candy, soda, pickles and alcoholic beverages. It is one of the most versatile, ancient, significant, medicinal, nutritional herbs with several ethnomedical values. This plant is recognised due to its therapeutic properties, including antibiotic, antimicrobial, antioxidant and anti-inflammatory effects [29]. Phenolic acids, diarylheptanoids, terpenoids and flavonoids are reported to exist in ginger rhizomes [30]. A list of 72 gingerols and diarylheptanoids derivatives from ginger rhizomes is presented in Asamenew et al. [31], and among these compounds, gingerol- and shogaol-related derivatives are the principal medicinally active components contributing to the characteristic pungent flavour of ginger together with essential oil major component, zingerone. These bioactive compounds have been shown in experiments to be effective for inflammatory diseases [32] and osteoarthritis [29], to help induce apoptosis in cancer cells [33] and to show anti-leukaemic effect [34]. Ginger has a great pharmaceutical potential.

Our survey of recent (2019) publications on Zingiberaceae in the Web-of-Science database, using "*Curcuma*" as keyword in titles (**Figure 2**), shows that *C. longa* (turmeric, saffron turmeric) is the single most researched *Curcuma* species. The results show that this species has received much attention in the area of pharmaceutical research and medicinal applications. Turmeric is commonly used as spice, dye, drug and cosmetics [35], but recent research efforts have further characterised its medicinal properties and have identified its biochemical components in high resolution and specificity. The genus *Curcuma* is rich in flavonoids, tannins, anthocyanin, phenolic compounds, oil, organic acids and inorganic compounds [36]. The biological activities of *Curcuma* have been attributed to the non-volatile ingredients of the rhizome, cucurminoids (e.g. curcumin), as well as to the volatile terpenoids [37]. Curcumin has been shown in experiments to have strong anti-inflammatory and antioxidant effects [29, 36]. The European Union has

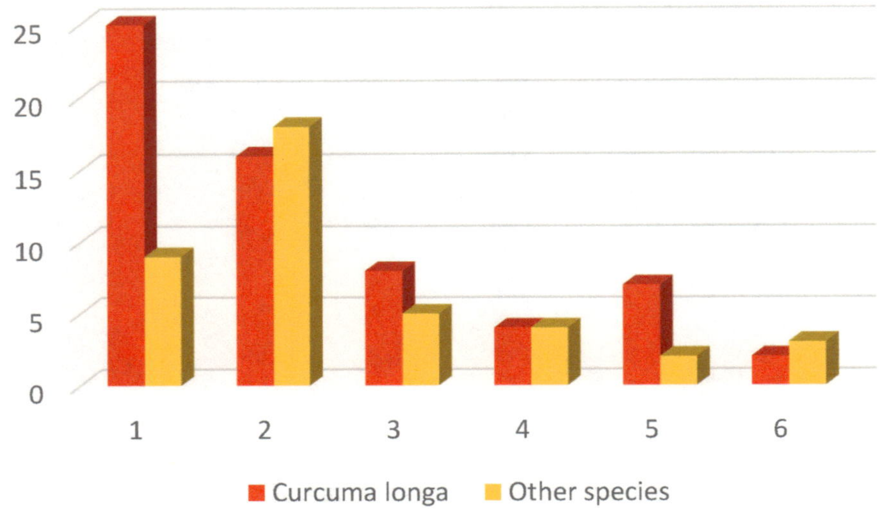

Figure 2.
Distribution of recent publications by research topics in 2019, obtained from web-of-science database (webofknowledge.com/WOS_), using the single keyword "Curcuma" in title. Research topics (x-axis): 1, medicinal properties and health benefits; 2, pharmaceutical, biochemical and molecular research; 3, food science and chemistry; 4, other technologies and industrial applications; 5, cultivation and agriculture; and 6, biodiversity, taxonomy, ecology and genetics. Y-axis: Percentages of the number of publications in 200 totals. Red columns include papers on Curcuma longa *(turmeric). Yellow columns include papers about all other* Curcuma *species, e.g.* C. zedoaria *(white turmeric, 7%),* C. caesia *(black turmeric, 5%),* C. xanthorrhiza *(Javanese ginger/turmeric, 5%),* C. amada *(mango ginger, 5%),* C. aromatica *(fragrant turmeric, 3%) and 17 other* Curcuma *species with less than 3% each.*

recommended the use of numerous medicinal plants for the treatment of gastrointestinal disorders, and among them are ginger root (*Z. officinale*) and turmeric root (*C. longa*) [38].

Some 23 other *Curcuma* species have recently been explored in search for new medicinal applications (**Figure 2**). The top five *Curcuma* species investigated are *C. zedoaria* (Christm.) Rosc. (white turmeric, native to South and Southeast Asia, cultivated in Thailand), *C. caesia* Roxb. (black turmeric, native to Northeast India, natural species of Thailand), *C. xanthorrhiza* Roxb. (Javanese ginger/turmeric, originated from Java island, cultivated in Thailand), *C. amada* Roxb. (mango ginger, originated from East India, natural species of Thailand) and *C. aromatica* Roxb. (fragrant turmeric, natural species of South Asia, cultivated in Thailand). Bioactive ingredients, including terpenes (more than 40 monoterpenes and sesquiterpenes), antioxidants flavonoids and phenolic compounds are present in all these species [39, 40]. Curcumin from *C. zedoaria*, as from *C. longa*, shows good anti-inflammatory effects [36]. Zederone and zedoarondiol, from rhizomes of En-Lueang (*Curcuma cf. amada*), show strong cytotoxicity in a leukaemic cell line and in peripheral blood mononuclear cells, as well as having antioxidant and haemolysis properties [41]. Dry extracts from rhizomes of *C. xanthorrhiza* and *C. zedoaria* have been shown to have anticancer and antiviral properties [42–44]. Furthermore, volatile oils extracted from leaves of *C. caesia* have broad antioxidant, anti-inflammatory and antimicrobial effects in vitro [45, 46]. In contrast to *C. longa*, many of the medicinal *Curcuma* species are not in large-scale cultivation, and this increases the risk of overharvesting of rhizomes from wild plants. The good news is that researchers are beginning to improve local cultivars and finding suitable methods of micropropagation of these *Curcuma* species, for example, *C. angustifolia* Roxb. [47].

4. The genus *Curcuma* in Thailand

Forty-five species are found in Thailand or almost 50% of the total species diversity of *Curcuma* worldwide (**Table 1**). At least 12 of these species are endemic to Thailand. New species have recently been described. For example, *C. saraburiensis* Boonma & Saensouk from Saraburi province, Central Thailand [48] and *C. putii* Maknoi & Jenjitt [49]. Several species of *Curcuma* are cultivated throughout Thailand for commercial purposes. The whole plant has economic values: the above-ground part of the plant bears attractive flowers that have been exported worldwide as cut flowers, such as Siam tulip (*C. alismatifolia*) and *C. parviflora* Wall. [50], whereas the below-ground rhizomes are harvested and sold in local markets for use as crude extracts in the traditional medicine or for the production of certified pharmaceutical products. Medicinal species, such as *C. comosa* Roxb., has received much attention in recent years for being a phytoestrogen-producing plant (e.g. [51, 52]). Products from rhizomes of *C. comosa* have been developed for use as an anti-inflammation remedy and for treatment of uterine abnormalities and ovarian hormone deficit [53, 54].

Species of *Curcuma* L.	2*n* chromosome number	Ploidy	Natural	Cultivated	References
C. aeruginosa Roxb.	63	Triploid		x	4, 6, 9
C. alismatifolia Gagnep.	32		x	x	9
C. amada Roxb.	42	Diploid	x		1, 2, 4, 9, 10
C. angustifolia Roxb.	42 (64)	Diploid	x		4, 6, 9, 10
C. aromatica Roxb.	42, 63, 86	Di-, tri-, tetraploid		x	1, 2, 3, 4, 6, 7, 9, 10
C. aurantiaca van Zijp	42	Diploid	x	x	4, 6, 9, 10
C. bella Maknoi*, K. Larsen & Sirirugsa**a**					
C. bicolor J.Mood & K. Larsen			x	x	
C. caesia Roxb.***b**	63	Triploid	x		9, 10
C. candida (Wall.) Techapr.***c**	42	Diploid	x		12
C. cochinchinensis Gagnep.			x		
C. comosa Roxb.	42, 63	Di-, triploid	x	x	5, 9, 11
C. ecomata Craib			x		
C. elata Roxb.***d**	63	Triploid		x	4, 5, 7, 9, 11
C. flaviflora S.Q.Tong	42	Diploid	x		7
C. glans K. Larsen & J. Mood			x		
C. glacillima Gagnep.	ca. 32		x		
C. hermandii Gagnep.	20		x	x	9
C. latifolia Roxb.	63, 84	Tri-, tetraploid	x	x	4, 5, 9, 11
C. leucorhiza Roxb.		Triploid		x	6,

Species of *Curcuma* L.	2*n* chromosome number	Ploidy	Natural	Cultivated	References
C. longa L.	63 (32, 48, 62-64)	Triploid		x	1, 2, 4, 6, 9, 10
C. maehongson C. Maknoi			x		
C. mangga Val.	42 (63)	Diploid		x	4, 9
C. nakornsawan C. Maknoi			x		
C. parviflora Wall.	28, 30, 32, 36, 42		x		9
C. petiolata Roxb.	42, 64	Di-, triploid	x	x	9, 10
C. pierreana Gagnep.			x		
C. putii Maknoi & Jenjitt.***e**					
C. ranong C.Maknoi			x		
C. rhabdota Sirirugsa & M. Newman	24		x	x	9
C. roscoceana Wall.	42	Diploid	x	x	4, 9
C. rubescens Roxb.	63	Triploid		x	9
C. rubrobracteata Skornickova, Sabu & Prasanth k.	63	Triploid	x		7
C. saraburi C.Maknoi			x		
C. saraburiensis Boonma & Saensouk***f**			x		
C. singularis Gagnep.	42		x		9
C. sparganiifolia Gagnep.			x	x	
C. stenochila Gagnep.			x		
C. tak C.Maknoi			x		
C. ubonratchani C.Maknoi			x		
C. viridiflora Roxb.			x		
C. woodii N.H.Xia & J. Chen***g**	42	Diploid			8
C. xanthorrhiza Roxb.	63	Triploid		x	3, 6, 7, 9, 10
C. zedoaria (Christm.) Rosc.	63, 64, 84, 105	Tri-, tetra- pentaploid		x	2, 4, 6, 9, 10, 11
C. cf. *Zedoaroides* Chaveer. & Tanee***h**	63	Triploid	x		11
Total number of taxa = 45			**33**	**19**	

**Species references: a, Maknoi et al. [55]; b, Puangpairote [56]; c, Jenjittikul and Larsen [57]; d, Larsen [6]; e, Maknoi et al. [49]; f, Boonma and Saensouk [48]; g, Chen et al. [58]; and h, Puangpairote et al. [59]. Chromosome/ploidy references: 1. Ramachandran [60]; 2. Ramachandran [61]; 3. eFlora [9]; 4. Leong-Skornikova et al. [10]; 5. Soontornchainaksaeng and Jenjitikul [51]; 6. Zaveska et al. [62]; 7. Chen et al. [63]; 8. Chen et al. [58]; 9. Puangpairote [56]; 10. Rice et al. [64]; 11. Puangpairote et al. [59]; 12. Nopporncharoenkul et al. [65].*

Table 1.
List of Curcuma *species found in Thailand, based on Maknoi [11] (except *), with* 2n *somatic chromosome number, ploidy level and distribution.*

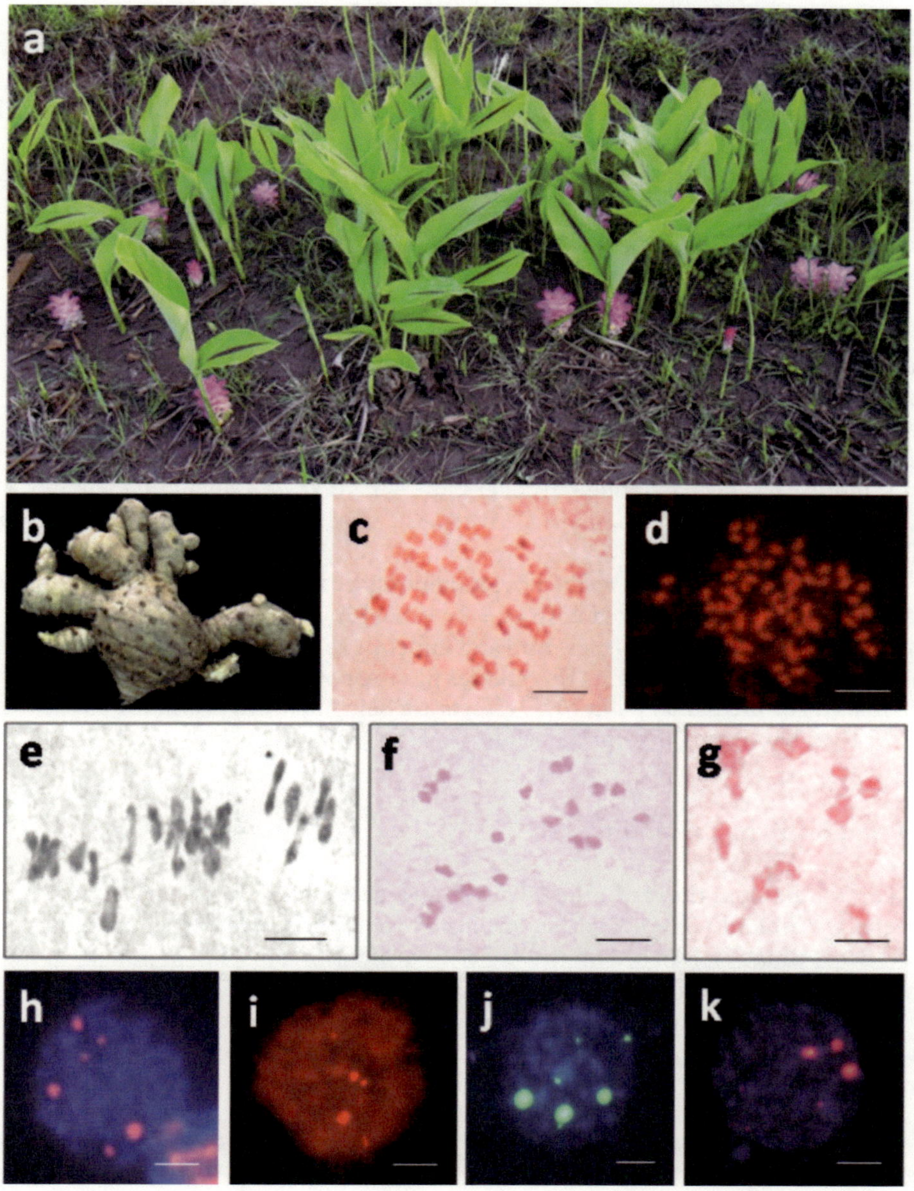

Figure 3.
Our own research work on selected Curcuma *species from Thailand. (a) Triploid* Curcuma comosa *plants, showing the above-ground part of the plant with 60–150-cm-tall leafy shoots and 15–32-cm-long inflorescences with short peduncle and dark pink flowers. (b) Rhizome of the triploid* Curcuma *sp.* "elata-latifolia"*. Typical rhizome of this species is ovoid-ellipsoid in shape and about (7–15) × (6–10) cm in size, with 2–7 lateral rhizomes, 2–12 cm long and up to 5 secondary lateral rhizomes. (c) Mitotic metaphase cell of* C. candida *showing diploid chromosome number 2n = 42. (d) Mitotic metaphase cell of* C. comosa *showing diploid chromosome number 2n = 42. (e) Male meiotic cell of the diploid* C. candida *showing normal chromosome pairing with 21 bivalents at metaphase-I. (f) Male meiotic cell of the triploid cytotype of* C. comosa *showing chromosome pairing at metaphase-I with 21 trivalents, indicating autotriploidy. (g) Male meiotic cell of the triploid* C. latifolia *showing irregular synapsis at metaphase-I chromosome pairing with 21 trivalents, indicating allotriploidy. (h) A mitotic interphase cell of the triploid cytotype of* C. comosa *showing three major sites of the 45S ribosomal genes, confirming triploidy in this species. (i) A mitotic interphase cell of the triploid cytotype of* C. comosa *showing three major sites of the 45S ribosomal genes, one large* C. comosa *marker site Cc1 and two smaller sites. (j) A mitotic interphase cell of the triploid cytotype of* C. elata *showing three major sites of the 45S ribosomal genes and three minor sites, confirming triploidy in this species. (k) A mitotic interphase cell of the triploid cytotype of* C. elata *showing three major sites of the 45S ribosomal genes, again confirming triploidy in this species. Scale bars represent 5 μm. References: (a–b) [51]; (c, e) [65]; (d, f–g) [59]; (h, j–k) [66]; and (i) [56].*

We have studied *C. comosa* and its related species, collectively called wan-chak-motluk in Thai language for its phytoestrogen properties. The plant produces bright colourful flowers in the form of inflorescences (**Figure 3a**). Its rhizomes are ovoid to ovate spheroidal in shape and about 8–15 cm in diameter (**Figure 3b**). Wan-chak-motluk belongs to three *Curcuma* species: *C. comosa*, *C. elata* Roxb. and *C. latifolia* Rosc. [51]. *Curcuma comosa* is recognised by its inflorescences with short peduncles (**Figure 3a**), whereas the other two species have long peduncles more suitable for flower arrangements. *Curcuma elata* and *C. latifolia* produce large and branchy rhizomes (**Figure 3b**).

Our chromosome number investigations have shown that the three wan-chak-motluk species can be further separated into five cultivars or cytotypes ([51]; see also **Table 1**): *C. comosa* has two cytotypes, diploid with $2n = 2x = 42$ (**Figure 3d**) and triploid with $2n = 3x = 63$ (**Figure 3f**); *C. elata* (and *C.* cf. "*elata-latifolia*") is triploid with $2n = 3x = 63$; but *C. latifolia* has two cytotypes, triploid with $2n = 3x = 63$ (**Figure 3g**) and tetraploid with $2n = 4x = 84$. The group of wan-chak-motluk has been extended to cover more Thai taxa [59], including triploid *C. caesia*, triploid *C.* cf. *zedoaroides* Chaveer. & Tanee and tetraploid *C.* cf. *zedoaria* (Christm.) Rosc.

We have also recently described cytotaxonomy of the white flowering *C. candida* (Wall.) Techapr., to be diploid with $2n = 2x = 42$ ([65]; **Figure 3c, e**). *C. candida* is a conservation-vulnerable species, rare and endemic to the Tenasserim Range bordering Thailand and Myanmar. As this species has the potential to be developed as an ornamental or medicinal plant [67], efforts are being made to promote cultivation rather than harvesting it from the wild.

5. Polyploidy in *Curcuma*

Our studies and those of others have shown that while most Thai *Curcuma* species are diploid ($2n = 42$), other species are polyploid (**Table 1**). This ploidy level determination is based on the meiotic chromosome pairing in pollen mother cells, i.e. a diploid plant shows 21 bivalents, resulting from a complete synapsis of homologous chromosomes at metaphase-I of the meiotic cell division (e.g. **Figure 3e**). Therefore, we have concluded that the base chromosome number for *Curcuma*, at least the Thai species investigated, to be 21 ($x = 21$), but we have also identified this as "secondary" base chromosome number, possibly deriving from three times primary base number $x = 7$ [59, 66]. Leong-Skornickova et al. [10] measured genome size of 51 Indian *Curcuma* taxa using flow cytometry and obtained chromosome counts from about one-third of the plants. They established that the base number was $x = 7$ for Indian *Curcuma* because all the $2n$ numbers in their study were multiples of seven, from hexaploids ($2n = 42$) up to 15-ploids. This $x = 7$ is most likely an ancestral base number of *Curcuma*. Most angiosperms, woody and herbaceous, are considered being ancient polyploids with the original base numbers $x = 6$ and $x = 7$ [68]. The major crop plants of the world are polyploid, for example, wheat, maize, potatoes, banana, cotton, oilseed rape and coffee beans, and most of these highly productive plants are ancient polyploids [69]. Therefore, in this context, all Thai *Curcuma* species (**Table 1**) are basically (ancient) polyploids, ranging from $2n = 42$ (primary hexaploid, secondary diploid) to $2n = 63$ (primary 9-ploid, secondary triploid) and $2n = 84$ (primary 12-ploid, secondary tetraploid). However, for the matter of consistency among our studies, we treat all Thai *Curcuma* taxa based on the secondary base number $x = 21$. This is in line with most other chromosome studies, whereby the meiotic analysis is used to determine ploidy levels, for example, the most cultivated turmeric species *C. longa* is triploid with $2n = 63$ [60, 64].

The genus *Curcuma* contains chromosome numbers spanning the full range of the family Zingiberaceae, from $2n = 20$ to 105 [10, 51, 59, 61, 63, 64, 70], but is characterised by chromosomes of particularly small sizes, usually less than 2 μm. A large number of *Curcuma* species (at least 25 species) have the diploid chromosome number $2n = 42$ (base number $x = 21$), several (ca. 12) species have $2n = 63$, and other numbers such as 20, 24, 32, 34, 84 and 105 have also been reported. Polyploidy is indeed very common in the ginger family Zingiberaceae.

Fluorescent in situ hybridization (FISH) mapping of the tandemly repeated 45S (18S–25S) ribosomal DNA on chromosomes of wan-chak-motluk supports the occurrence of triploidy among the species and cytotypes with $2n = 63$ [66]. Sets of three ribosomal FISH signals (loci) are apparent in the triploid *C. comosa* (**Figure 3h**, **i**) and the triploid *C. elata* (**Figure 3j**, **k**). In addition, the meiotic figure obtained from the triploid cytotype of *C. comosa* comprises of 21 trivalents; each is a pairing of three homologous chromosomes (**Figure 3f**). Cytogenetic characteristics of triploidy have been observed in other *Curcuma* species, such as *C. longa* [60] and *C. zedoaria* [71].

This triploidization is likely to be the outcome of hybridization between unreduced ($2n$) and normal ($1n$) gametes within or between the diploid populations. Such mechanism has been well documented [72, 73]. In Zingiberaceae, multiple occurrences of triploid formation have been shown in the ornamental ginger genus *Globba* L. from Southeast Asia, based on molecular phylogenetic analysis of both chloroplast and nuclear genes [74]. The situation with *Curcuma*—wan-chak-motluk—is similar to that of *Globba* in that tetraploids ($2n = 84$) are extremely rare (**Table 1**) and the triploids are variable both morphologically and cytogeographically [51]. The molecular study by Zaveska et al. [75] has shown that in *Curcuma*, the genus of palaeopolyploid origin, its evolution is most likely driven by hybridization and polyploidization.

Once a triploid has arisen, it could easily survive because *Curcuma*, like other genera in Zingiberaceae, reproduces predominantly by vegetative means, i.e. the plants often propagate by rhizomes and numerous bulbils produced on the inflorescence. In the context of cultivation and utilisation of wan-chak-motluk, triploid cultivars (with 2n = 63) are indeed very popular among the growers, for example, for having larger rhizomes. We have also found that triploid and tetraploid plants do have proportionally larger genome sizes compared with the diploid plants [59]. Polyploidization in plants often increases cell size as well as growth rates, giving rise to plant phenotypes having higher physiological capacity and productivity [76]. Increasing the ploidy level is known to be positively correlated with plant production, both biomass and yield [69]. Furthermore, polyploids are often said to have a broader ecological tolerance than their diploid progenitors [77]. This is thought to be due to the effects of increased heterozygosity providing metabolic flexibility to cope with wider arrays of conditions [76]. In addition, the advantages of having more copies of the genes should allow polyploids to thrive in environments that pose challenges to their diploid progenitors [78]. In Zingiberaceae, triploids are highly successful in cultivation, mainly due to their productive rhizomes. In natural environments, triploids may be superior as a likely result of the plant's fitness as described above. *Curcuma* triploids are indeed common and widespread over a vast geographical range throughout Asia [9, 10, 62, 63, 70, 71]. Future studies combining cytogenomics, genetics, physiology and ecology should shed light onto the underlying physiological mechanism and its genetic basis of such gains in polyploidy.

6. Conclusion

The most widely cultivated plants belong to the two largest genera of this family, the ginger genus (*Zingiber*) and the turmeric genus (*Curcuma*). They are also the best researched plants from this family, and the most researched topics concern medicinal properties and health benefits, pharmaceutical, biochemical and molecular characterisation, as well as applications in food science and technology. The present study identifies numerous polyploid species in the turmeric genus (*Curcuma*) from Thailand. In particular, triploid species and/or cultivars are popular for a large-scale cultivation. The plants are easily propagated via underground rhizomes, which are also the part of the plant that contains bioactive compounds with medicinal properties. Rhizomes of triploid cultivars are bigger than those of the diploid, wild relatives and thus are more economically valuable. Triploids are also the most adaptable plants in diverse environments. On the other hand, the overharvesting of wild plants, in search for novel or better bioactive compounds, poses a serious risk of species extinction. Cytogenetic research, such as that presented here, can provide useful information for both types of activities, i.e. in the plant improvement for cultivation and in the conservation of natural biodiversity.

Acknowledgements

This work was supported by Mahidol University and University of Iceland. We appreciate the contribution in taxonomic identification of plant materials from Dr. Thaya Jenjittikul of Mahidol University. We thank both Dr. Tidarat Puangpairote from Prince of Songkla University and PhD student of Mahidol University, Nattapon Nopporncharoenkul, for their accurate cytogenetic work on Zingiberaceae of Thailand.

Author details

Kesara Anamthawat-Jónsson[1] and Puangpaka Umpunjun[2*]

1 Institute of Life and Environmental Sciences, University of Iceland, Reykjavík, Iceland

2 Department of Plant Science, Faculty of Science, Mahidol University, Bangkok, Thailand

*Address all correspondence to: puangpaka.ump@mahidol.ac.th

References

[1] eFloras. 20. Zingiberaceae Lindley. In: Flora of China. Vol. 24. St. Louis, 15 MO/Cambridge, MA: Missouri Botanical Garden/Harvard University Herbaria; 2020. p. 322. Available from: http://www.efloras.org [Accessed: 23 February 2020]

[2] Wu DL, Larsen K. Zingiberaceae. In: Wu ZY, Raven P, Hong DY, editors. Flora of China. Vol. 24. Beijing, China/St. Louis, MO: Science Press/ Missouri Botanical Garden Press; 2000. pp. 322-377

[3] Larsen K, Larsen S. Gingers of Thailand. Chiang Mai: Queen Sirikit Botanic Garden; 2006

[4] Leong-Skornickova J, Newman M. Gingers of Cambodia, Laos and Vietnam. Singapore: Singapore Botanic Gardens; 2015

[5] Saensouk S. Endemic and rare plants of gingers family in Thailand. Khon Kaen University Research Journal. 2011;**16**:306-330

[6] Larsen K. A preliminary checklist of the Zingiberaceae of Thailand. Thai Forest Bulletin (Botany). 1996;**24**:35-49

[7] eFloras. 1. *Zingiber* Miller. In: Flora of China. Vol. 24. St. Louis, 15 MO/ Cambridge, MA: Missouri Botanical Garden/Harvard University Herbaria; 2020. p. 323. [Internet]. Available from: http://www.efloras.org [Accessed: 23 February 2020]

[8] WCSP. World Checklist of Selected Plant Families [Internet]. Kew: Royal Botanic Gardens; 2020. Available from: http://wcsp.science.kew.org/ [Accessed: 23 February 2020]

[9] eFloras. 11. *Curcuma* Linnaeus. In: Flora of China [Internet]. Vol. 24. St. Louis, 15 MO/Cambridge, MA: Missouri Botanical Garden/Harvard University Herbaria; 2020. p. 359. Available from: http://www.efloras.org [Accessed: 23 February 2020]

[10] Leong-Skornickova J, Sida O, Jarolimova V, Sabu M, Fer T, Travnicek P, et al. Chromosome numbers and genome size variation in Indian species of *Curcuma* (Zingiberaceae). Annals of Botany. 2007;**100**:505-526

[11] Maknoi C. Taxonomy and phylogeny of the genus *Curcuma L.* (Zingiberaceae) with particular reference to its occurrence in Thailand [PhD thesis]. Thailand: Prince of Songkla University; 2006

[12] Walther G-R, Post E, Convey P, Menzel A, Parmesan C, et al. Ecological responses to recent climate change. Nature. 2002;**416**:389-395

[13] Laurance WF, Sayer J, Cassman KG. Agricultural expansion and its impacts on tropical nature. Trends in Ecology & Evolution. 2014;**29**:107-116

[14] Newbold T, Hudson LN, Hill SLL, Contu S, Lysenko I, et al. Global effects of land use on local terrestrial biodiversity. Nature. 2015;**520**:45-50

[15] Romand-Monnier F, Contu S. *Curcuma caulina*. In: The IUCN Red List of Threatened Species. 2013. DOI: 10.2305/IUCN.UK.2013-1.RLTS. T44392545A44510728.en [Accessed: 23 February 2020]

[16] Olander SB. *Curcuma colorata*. In: The IUCN Red List of Threatened Species. 2019. DOI: 10.2305/IUCN.UK.2019-3.RLTS. T117308749A124281530.en [Accessed: 23 February 2020]

[17] Romand-Monnier F. *Curcuma coriacea*. In: The IUCN Red List of Threatened Species. 2013. DOI:

10.2305/IUCN.UK.2013-1.RLTS.T44393421A44507719.en [Accessed: 23 February 2020]

[18] Leong-Skornickova J, Souvannakhoummane K, Tran HD. *Curcuma corniculata*. In: The IUCN Red List of Threatened Species. 2019. DOI: 10.2305/IUCN.UK.2019-3.RLTS.T125297777A125297800.en [Accessed: 23 February 2020]

[19] Leong-Skornickova J. *Curcuma prasina*. In: The IUCN Red List of Threatened Species. 2019. DOI: 10.2305/IUCN.UK.2019-3.RLTS.T125297897A125297901.en [Accessed: 23 February 2020]

[20] Tran HD, Leong-Skornickova J. *Curcuma sahuynhensis*. In: The IUCN Red List of Threatened Species. 2019. DOI: 10.2305/IUCN.UK.2019-3.RLTS.T131724352A131724370.en [Accessed: 23 February 2020]

[21] Leong-Skornickova J, Tran HD, Newman MF, Dinh Quang D. *Curcuma vitellina*. In: The IUCN Red List of Threatened Species. 2019. DOI: 10.2305/IUCN.UK.2019-3.RLTS.T201889A132688601.en [Accessed: 23 February 2020]

[22] Sabu M. *Curcuma bhatii*. In: The IUCN Red List of Threatened Species. 2019. DOI: 10.2305/IUCN.UK.2019-3.RLTS.T117308352A124281490.en [Accessed: 23 February 2020]

[23] Leong-Skornickova J. *Curcuma leonidii*. In: The IUCN Red List of Threatened Species. 2019. DOI: 10.2305/IUCN.UK.2019-3.RLTS.T131774861A131774866.en. [Accessed: 23 February 2020]

[24] Leong-Skornickova J, Tran HD. *Curcuma newmanii*. In: The IUCN Red List of Threatened Species. 2019. DOI: 10.2305/IUCN.UK.2019-3.RLTS.T132967025A132967030.en [Accessed: 23 February 2020]

[25] Leong-Skornickova J, Tran HD. *Curcuma pygmaea*. In: The IUCN Red List of Threatened Species. 2019. DOI: 10.2305/IUCN.UK.2019-3.RLTS.T131774887A131774892.en [Accessed: 23 February 2020]

[26] Leong-Skornickova J, Tran HD, Newman M, Lamxay V, Bouamanivong S. *Curcuma supraneeana*. In: The IUCN Red List of Threatened Species. 2019. DOI: 10.2305/IUCN.UK.2019-3.RLTS.T201917A132691416.en. [Accessed: 23 February 2020]

[27] Sabu M. *Curcuma vamana*. In: The IUCN Red List of Threatened Species. 2019. DOI: 10.2305/IUCN.UK.2019-3.RLTS.T117310982A124281770.en [Accessed: 23 February 2020]

[28] Ravindran PN, Nirmal Babu K. Ginger: The Genus Zingiber. CRC Press; 2005. pp. 576

[29] Panda SK, Kumari KL, Adhikari L, Sahu PK, Pal A. A review on clinical efficacy of traditional plants on osteoarthritis. International Journal of Pharmaceutical Sciences and Research. 2019;**10**:4040-4053

[30] Gu C, Howell K, Dunshea FR, Suleria HAR. LC-ESI-QTOF/MS characterization of phenolic acids and flavonoids in polyphenol-rich fruits and vegetables and their potential antioxidant activities. Antioxidants. 2019;**8**. article 405

[31] Asamenew G, Kim H-W, Lee M-K, Lee S-H, Kim YJ, et al. Characterization of phenolic compounds from normal ginger (*Zingiber officinale* Rosc.) and black ginger (*Kaempferia parviflora* wall.) using UPLC-DAD-QToF-MS. European Food Research and Technology. 2019;**245**:653-665

[32] Ara T, Koide M, Kitamura H, Sogowa N. Effects of shokyo (*Zingiberis Rhizoma*) and kankyo (*Zingiberis Processum Rhizoma*) on prostaglandin

E2 production in lipopolysaccharide-treated mouse macrophage RAW264.7 cells. PeerJ. 2019;7. article e7725

[33] Gan HY, Zhang YQ, Zhou QY, Zheng LR, Xie XF, et al. Zingerone induced caspase-dependent apoptosis in MCF-7 cells and prevents 7,12-dimethylbenz(a) anthracene-induced mammary carcinogenesis in experimental rats. Journal of Biochemical and Molecular Toxicology. 2019;**33**. article e22387

[34] Babasheikhali SR, Rahgozar S, Mohammadi M. Ginger extract has anti-leukemia and anti-drug resistant effects on malignant cells. Journal of Cancer Research and Clinical Oncology. 2019;**145**:1987-1998

[35] Ravindran PN, Nirmal BK, Sivaraman K. Turmeric: The Genus Curcuma (Medicinal and Aromatic Plants-Industrial Profiles). Abingdon: Taylor and Francis Group; 2007. pp. 484

[36] Ayati Z, Ramezani M, Amiri MS, Moghada AT, Rahimi H, Abdollahzade A, et al. Ethnobotany, phytochemistry and traditional uses of *Curcuma* spp. and pharmacological profiles of two important species (*C. longa* and *C. zedoaria*): Review. Current Pharmaceutical Design. 2019;**25**:871-935

[37] Dosoky NS, Satyal P, Setzer WS. Variations in the volatile compositions of *Curcuma* species. Food. 2019;**8**. article 53

[38] Thumann TA, Pferschy-Wenzig E-M, Moissl-Eichinger C, Bauer R. The role of gut microbiota for the activity of medicinal plants traditionally used in the European Union for gastrointestinal disorders. Journal of Ethnopharmacology. 2019;**245**. article 112153

[39] Akter J, Hossain M a, Takara K, Islam MZ, Hou D-X. Antioxidant activity of different species and varieties of turmeric (*Curcuma* spp.): Isolation of active compounds. Comparative Biochemistry and Physiology C: Toxicology & Pharmacology. 2019;**215**:9-17

[40] De B, Karak S, Das S, Begum S, Gupta P, De Pradhan I, et al. Profiling non-polar terpenes of rhizomes for distinguishing some Indian *Curcuma* species. Journal of Applied Research on Medicinal and Aromatic Plants. 2019;**13**. article UNSP 100207

[41] Anuchapreeda S, Khumpirapang N, Chiampanichayakul S, Nirachonkul W, Saiai A, Usuki T, et al. Characterization and biological properties of zederone and zedoarondiol from rhizomes of en-Lueang (*Curcuma* cf. *amada*). Natural Product Communications. 2018;**13**:1615-1618

[42] Lourembam RM, Yadav AS, Kundu GC, Mazumder PB. *Curcuma zedoaria* (Christm.) roscoe inhibits proliferation of MDA-MB231 cells via caspase-cascade apoptosis. Oriental Pharmacy and Experimental Medicine. 2019;**19**:235-241

[43] Sufiawati I, Gunawan I, Wijala I, Rusdiana T, Subranas A. Reduction of salivary tumor necrosis factor alpha levels in response to magic mouthwash with *Curcuma xanthorrhiza* in cancer patients undergoing chemotherapy. Journal of Research in Pharmacy. 2019;**23**:55-61

[44] Wahyuni TS, Permatasari AA, Widiandani T, Fuad A, Widyawaruyani A, Aoki-Uysubo C, et al. Antiviral activities of *Curcuma* genus against hepatitis C virus. Natural Product Communications. 2018;**13**:1570-1582

[45] Borah A, Paw M, Gogoi R, Loying R, Sarma N, Munda S, et al. Chemical composition, antioxidant, anti-inflammatory, anti-microbial and in-vitro cytotoxic efficacy of essential oil of *Curcuma caesia* Roxb. Leaves:

An endangered medicinal plant of north East India. Industrial Crops and Products. 2019;**129**:448-454

[46] Deeki LT, Manivannan SJ, Sujata U, Biswajit RG. Targeting metabolic profiling of black turmeric (*Curcuma caesia* Roxb.) accessions for industrially important compounds. Research Journal of Biotechnology. 2019;**14**:24-28

[47] Jena S, Ray A, Sahoo A, Sahoo S, Kar B, Panda PC, et al. High-frequency clonal propagation of *Curcuma angustifolia* ensuring genetic fidelity of micropropagated plants. Plant Cell, Tissue and Organ Culture. 2018;**135**:473-486

[48] Boonma T, Saensouk S. *Curcuma saraburiensis* (Zingiberaceae), a new species from Thailand. Taiwania. 2019;**64**:245-248

[49] Maknoi C, Ruchisansakul S, Jenjittikul T. *Curcuma putti* (Zingiberaceae), a new species from Thailand. Annales Botanici Fennici. 2019;**56**:351-353

[50] Khumkratok S, Boontiang K, Chutichudet P, Pramaul P. Geographical distributions and ecology of ornamental *Curcuma* (Zingiberaceae) in North-Eastern Thailand. Pakistan Journal of Biological Sciences. 2012;**15**:929-939

[51] Soontornchainaksaeng P, Jenjittikul T. Chromosome number variation of phytoestrogen-producing *Curcuma* (Zingiberaceae) from Thailand. Journal of Natural Medicines. 2010;**64**:370-377

[52] Thongon N, Boonmuen N, Suksen K, Wichit P, Chairoungdua A, et al. Selective Estrogen receptor modulator (SERM)-like activities of diarylheptanoid, a phytoestrogen from *Curcuma comosa*, in breast cancer cells, pre-osteoblast cells, and rat uterine tissues. Journal of Agricultural and Food Chemistry. 2017;**65**:3490-3496

[53] Jaipakdee N, Limpongsa E, Sripanidkulchai B, Piyachaturawat P. Preparation of *Curcuma comosa* tablets using liquisolid techniques: In vitro and in vivo evaluation. International Journal of Pharmaceutics. 2018;**553**:157-168

[54] Tabboon P, Tantiyasawasdikul S, Sripanidkulchai B. Quality and stability assessment of commercial products containing phytoestrogen diarylheptanoids from *Curcuma comosa*. Industrial Crops and Products. 2019;**134**:216-224

[55] Maknoi C, Sirirugsa P, Larsen K. *Curcuma bella* (Zingiberaceae), a new species from Thailand. Thai Journal of Botany. 2011;**3**:121-124

[56] Puangpairote T. Genomic characterization of phytoestrogen-producing curcuma in Thailand [PhD thesis]. Thailand: Mahidol University; 2015

[57] Jenjittikul T, Larsen K. *Kaempferia candida* wall. (Zingiberaceae), a new record for Thailand. Thai Forest Bulletin (Botany). 2000;**28**:45-49

[58] Chen J, Lindstrom AJ, Xia NH. *Curcuma woodii* (Zingiberaceae), a new species from Thailand. Phytotaxa. 2015;**227**:75-82

[59] Puangpairote T, Maknoi C, Jenjittikul T, Anamthawat-Jónsson K, Soontornchainaksaeng P. Natural triploidy in phyto-oestrogen producing *Curcuma* species and cultivars from Thailand. Euphytica. 2016;**208**:47-61

[60] Ramachandran K. Chromosome numbers in the genus *Curcuma* Linn. Current Science India. 1961;**30**:194-196

[61] Ramachandran K. Chromosome numbers in Zingiberaceae. Cytologia. 1969;**34**:213-221

[62] Zaveska E, Fer T, Sida O, Leong-Skornickova J, Sabu M, Marhold K.

Genetic diversity patterns in *Curcuma* reflects differences in genome size. Botanical Journal of the Linnean Society. 2011;**165**:388-401

[63] Chen J, Xia N, Zhao J, Chen J, Henny R. Chromosome numbers and ploidy levels of Chinese *Curcuma* species. Horticultural Science. 2013;**48**:525-530

[64] Rice A, Glick L, Abadi S, Einhorn M, Kopelman NM, et al. The chromosome counts database (CCDB)—A community resource of plant chromosome numbers. New Phytologist. 2015;**206**:19-26

[65] Nopporncharoenkul N, Jenjittikul T, Chuenboonngarm N, Anamthawat-Jónsson K, Umpunjun P. Cytogenetic verification of *Curcuma candida* (Zingiberaceae) from Thailand and Myanmar. Thai Forest Bulletin (Botany). 2020;**48**:7-17

[66] Soontornchainaksaeng P, Anamthawat-Jónsson K. Ribosomal FISH mapping reveals hybridity in phyto-oestrogen producing *Curcuma* species from Thailand. Plant Systematics and Evolution. 2011;**292**:41-49

[67] Picheansoonthon C, Koonterm S. Notes on the genus *Kaempferia L.* (Zingiberaceae) in Thailand. Journal of Thai Traditional and Alternative Medicine. 2008;**6**:27-51

[68] Stebbins GL. Chromosomal Evolution in Higher Plants. Bristol, UK: J. W. Arrowsmith Ltd; 1971

[69] Leitch AR, Leitch IJ. Perspective—Genomic plasticity and the diversity of polyploidy plants. Science. 2008;**320**:481-483

[70] Sirisawad T, Sirirugsa P, Suwanthada C, Apavatjrut P. Investigation of chromosome numbers in 20 taxa of *Curcuma*. In: Chantaranothai P, Larsen K, Sirirugsa P, Simpson D, editors. Proceedings of the 3rd Symposium on the Family Zingiberaceae; Khon Kaen University, Thailand. 2003. pp. 54-62

[71] Islam MA, Meister A, Schubert V, Kloppstech K, Esch E. Genetic diversity and cytogenetic analysis in *Curcuma zedoaria* (Christm.) roscoe from Bangladesh. Genetic Resources and Crop Evolution. 2007;**54**:149-156

[72] Leitch IJ, Bennett MD. Polyploidy in angiosperms. Trends in Plant Science. 1997;**2**:470-476

[73] Ramsey J, Schemske DW. Pathways, mechanisms, and rates of polyploidy formation in flowering plants. Annual Review of Ecology, Evolution, and Systematics. 1998;**29**:467-501

[74] Takano A, Okada H. Multiple occurrence of triploid formation in *Globba* (Zingiberaceae) from molecular evidence. Plant Systematics and Evolution. 2002;**230**:143-159

[75] Zaveska E, Fer T, Sida O, Krak K, Marhold K, Leong-Skornickova J. Hybridization among distantly related species: Examples from the polyploid genus *Curcuma* (Zingiberaceae). Molecular Phylogenetics and Evolution. 2016;**100**:303-321

[76] Otto SP, Whitton J. Polyploid incidence and evolution. Annual Review of Genetics. 2000;**34**:401-437

[77] Levin DA. Polyploidy and novelty in flowering plants. The American Naturalist. 1983;**122**:1-25

[78] Madlung A. Polyploidy and its effect on evolutionary success: Old questions revisited with new tools. Heredity. 2013;**110**:99-104

Chapter 9

Maize Chromosome Abnormalities and Breakage-Fusion-Bridge Cycles in Callus Cultures

Margarida L.R. Aguiar-Perecin, Janay A. Santos-Serejo, José R. Gardingo and Mateus Mondin

Abstract

The maize karyotype was first characterized by the observation of pachytene chromosomes. The somatic chromosomes were identified by C-banding and FISH with repetitive DNA sequences. C-banding was useful for the identification of chromosome abnormalities in callus cultures. In the present review, we focus on the involvement of heterochromatic knobs on the occurrence of chromosome abnormalities in callus cultures. In a previous work we detected anaphase bridges resulting from delayed chromatid separation at knob regions and typical bridges derived from dicentric chromatids in cultures. The analysis of altered chromosomes showed they were derived from a chromatid-type breakage-fusion-bridge (BFB) cycle. Fluorescent in situ hybridization (FISH) showed signals of telomere sequences in the broken chromosome arm, thus giving evidence of de novo telomere formation on the broken chromosome end. Further observations of long- and short-term cultures have shown the presence of chromosome alterations derived from BFB cycles followed by chromosome healing. Additionally, the occurrence of unequal crossing over in a knob region was observed in callus culture. These results are of interest for studies on the mechanisms of chromosome alterations during evolution.

Keywords: maize, heterochromatic knobs, chromosomal rearrangements, callus culture, breakage-fusion-bridge cycle, unequal crossing over

1. Introduction

Maize is an important crop plant and model organism. The maize karyotype was first characterized by the observation of pachytene chromosomes obtained from pollen mother cells, since the pioneering work by McClintock [1]. The early cytological maps were constructed based on the identification of chromosome relative lengths, arm ratios, heterochromatin patterns, prominent chromomeres, and nuclear organizer region [2–5]. Structures containing heterochromatin were described: heterochromatic knobs, centromeric heterochromatin, B chromosomes, abnormal chromosome 10, and nucleolus organizer region localized on chromosome 6 [6]. Chromosome abnormalities were detected in several investigations, and collections were organized containing reciprocal translocations (A-A translocations), B-A translocations (interchanges between B chromosome and arms of the A set), inversions, and trisomics, available at the Maize Genetics Cooperation

Stock Center [7] (www.maizegdb.org). These materials have been important tools for gene mapping.

The somatic chromosomes were identified by the C-banding procedure which was useful for the identification of chromosomal abnormalities in callus cultures [8–10]. The unequivocal identification of the somatic chromosomes is difficult due to their degree of condensation, and the use of the C-banding procedure was supplemented by an analysis of pachytene chromosomes of the lines from which callus cultures were derived. C-bands correspond to knobs visualized on meiotic chromosomes [11].

The characterization of meiotic and somatic chromosomes was improved by fluorescence in situ hybridization (FISH) using as probes repeated DNA sequences and genes, thus allowing the study of the molecular structure of chromosome components, such as centromere, neocentromere, B chromosome heterochromatic knobs, and gene mapping [12–20].

The maize chromosome structure has been extensively reviewed [21–25]. In the present review, we focus on the involvement of heterochromatic knobs on the occurrence of chromosome abnormalities in maize callus cultures. The size and number of knobs are variable, and they may be present in each of the 10 chromosomes of the complement at fixed positions in modern maize and its relatives, including species of *Zea* (teosintes) and *Tripsacum* [26, 27]. Knobs were mapped on the meiotic chromosomes [2, 3, 5], and recently they were mapped relative to the maize reference genome assembly [19]. Knobs are composed primarily of two tandemly repeated sequences, the 180-bp knob repeat and the 350-bp TR-1 element or a mixture of both [13, 17, 19]. Knobs also contain retrotransposons [28, 29].

One genetic effect attributed to knobs is their influence on recombination [6, 19], and it was revealed that knobs in heterozygous condition can reduce local recombination [19]. Another interesting genetic effect of knobs is their activity as neocentromeres resulting in meiotic drive. This meiotic event is a mechanism by which regions of the genome are preferentially transmitted to the progeny. In maize, meiotic drive is due to an uncommon form of chromosome 10, the abnormal chromosome 10 (Ab 10). In the presence of this chromosome, the knobs of other chromosomes are converted into motile neocentromeres. Thus the knobbed chromosomes preferentially segregate during female meiosis [30, 31]. The origin of maize polymorphism, including size and number, has been discussed in several reports, and it was proposed that meiotic drive was responsible for the evolution of knobs [32]. Recently, a cluster of eight genes on Ab10 was identified, called *Kinesin driver* (*Kindr*) complex, which are required for both neocentromere motility and preferential transmission. It was revealed that Kindr is a strong minus-end-directed motor that interacts specifically with neocentromeres containing 180-bp knob repeats [33].

The effect of knobs on chromosome break and origin of abnormalities in maize callus culture is presented in this review.

2. Chromosome abnormalities in maize callus culture

2.1 Heterochromatin involvement in chromosome breakage

Callus culture is an important step for genetic transformation in plants. The identification of maize genotypes showing high ability to form embryogenic callus type II (friable) and regenerate plants has progressed since the report by Green and Phillips [34]. The genotypes identified since then were adapted to temperate regions [35], and maize genotypes of tropical and subtropical origin have also been shown to produce friable type II calli capable to develop somatic embryogenesis [36–38].

Various studies have shown the occurrence of cytogenetic and genetic variability in plants regenerated from maize callus cultures [39, 40]. This so-called somaclonal variation [41] is undesirable when genetic stability is required, but interesting for the study of mechanisms that give rise to chromosome abnormalities. Chromosome breakage associated with heterochromatin was shown in several plant callus cultures [8–10, 42–48].

Breakpoints involved in chromosome abnormalities associated with heterochromatin were previously detected in maize regenerated plants. The analysis of pachytene chromosomes of these plants revealed that most breakpoints were localized in chromosomes bearing a knob. The authors hypothesized that late-replicating heterochromatin would replicate later in tissue culture, giving origin to bridges in anaphases and occurrence of breakage between the knob and centromere [47]. This would explain the presence of knobs in chromosomes involved in abnormalities observed in regenerated plants. The authors identified in meiotic cells alterations in chromosome structure, such as translocations, intercalary deficiencies, and heteromorphic pairs in 91 of 189 plants regenerated from callus cultures originated from an Oh43-A188 genetic background [47].

2.2 Breakage-fusion-bridge cycle in callus culture and de novo telomere formation

The first reports on breakage-fusion-bridge (BFB) cycles were made by McClintock [49, 50]. In investigations on the behavior in successive nuclear divisions of a chromosome broken at meiosis, it was shown that the chromatid type of BFB cycle initiated by broken chromosome ends occurs in gametophyte mitoses and in the endosperm. In the zygote the broken chromosome ends heal. BFB cycles have also been observed in other species including wheat (*Triticum aestivum*), in which reverse tandem duplications were observed [51]. The chromatid-type BFB cycle initiated in meiosis continued through pollen mitoses and in early endosperm divisions, but did not continue in embryo mitoses.

Investigations of mitotic cells in maize callus cultures detected anaphase bridges resulting in delayed separation at knob regions and typical bridges originated from dicentric chromatids. The observation of C-banded anaphases showed that the chromatids were held together at C-band sites (corresponding to knob) [8]. Typical bridges with and without C-bands were observed. These events were interpreted as derived from a chromatid type of BFB cycle initiated by chromatids that were broken during the primary event.

The analysis of abnormalities in chromosomes 7 and 9 of maize callus cultures gave evidence of their origin from BFB cycles [8–10]. As illustration, we show here the mechanism that would have originated these abnormalities. The callus culture was induced from a hybrid between two sister inbred lines derived from a tropical maize variety (Jac Duro [JD]). These JD lines possessed the same knob composition: K6 L2, K6 L3, K7S, K7L, K8 L1, K8 L2, and K9S [8, 20]. K refers to knob, the number identifies the chromosome, and S refers to short arm and L to long arm. Numbers 1, 2, and 3 refers to knob positions, according to the literature [27]. Thus, chromosome 7 possessed large knobs on both arms, and chromosome 9 had a very large knob on the short arm. Therefore, these chromosomes were more prone to suffer alterations.

An abnormal chromosome 7 carrying two knobs on the short arm was observed in metaphases of a callus culture designed 3–57. This abnormality was interpreted as being a deficiency-duplication (Df-Dp) derived from a BFB cycle and healing of the broken arm, for it was observed in various cells of the culture [8]. **Figure 1** [9, 25] shows the mechanism that would have originated this aberration. The two knobs on the short arm would bear a deficiency in the terminal region (RTD). Therefore this abnormal chromosome 7 possessed reverse tandem duplications of these knobs and of a segment designated “b.”

This chromosome 7 carrying a deficiency on K7S and duplications of the knob and of a “b” segment (Df-Dp7) was stable in culture and was transmitted to regenerated plants. Thus, R_0 plants regenerated from the 3–57 culture were heterozygous for this chromosome alteration. R_1 and R_2 plants were recovered and analyzed. Homozygotes for normal chromosome 7 and heterozygotes for the Df-Dp7 were detected. Plants homozygous for the Df-Dp7 were not recovered. Presumably, seeds carrying homozygotes were not viable. **Figure 2A** [9, 25] shows a metaphase of a

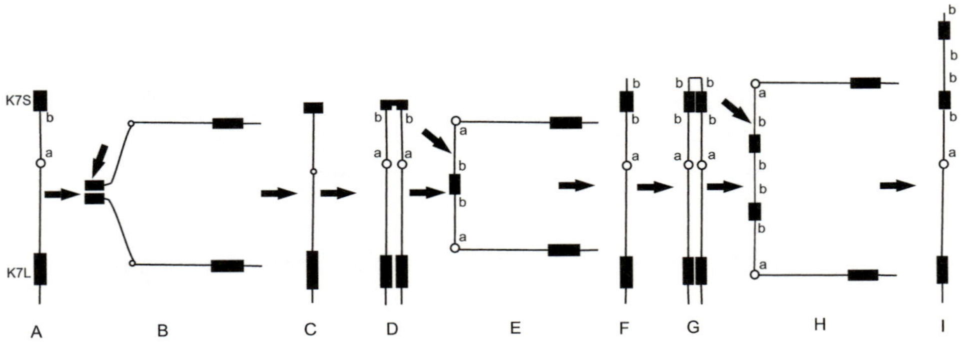

Figure 1.
BFB cycle that would give rise to chromosome 7 bearing a deficiency and duplication (Df-Dp) showing normal chromosome (A); anaphase with delayed separating chromatids and breakage at K7S (B); chromatid with a deficient K7S (C), fused after replication (D); breakage at anaphase (E); chromatid with duplication of the “b” segment (F), fused at broken ends (G); anaphase bridge and breakage (H); resulting chromatid with two knobs and reverse tandem duplications (RTD) of the “b” segment. Arrows at anaphases indicate breakpoints [9, 25].

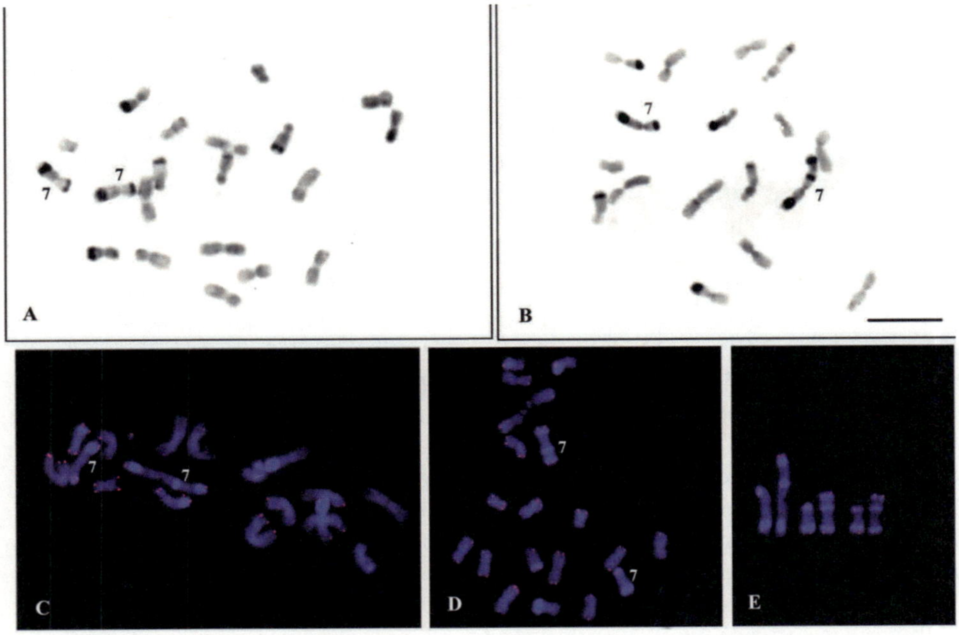

Figure 2.
Somatic chromosomes of R_1 plants derived from the 3–57 culture. C-banded mitotic metaphases homozygous for normal chromosome 7 showing knobs (C-bands) on the long and short arms (A); heterozygote for the Df-Dp chromosome 7 with two knobs; telomeric FISH signals on early and full metaphases (C, D); homologous pairs of chromosome 7 [9, 25].

regenerated plant homozygous for normal chromosome 7, and **Figure 2B** shows a metaphase of a plant heterozygous for the aberration. The distal knob (K7S) is subterminal, for there is a tiny terminal euchromatic segment on the short arm.

Fluorescent in situ hybridization (FISH) using the telomeric sequence $(TTTAGGG)_6$ showed signals in all the somatic chromosomes of the regenerated plants, including the Df-Dp7 chromosome (**Figure 2C–E**) [9, 25]. This result gives evidence of telomere healing at the end of the broken short arm. In these DAPI-stained metaphases, bands corresponding to the knobs could be clearly visualized. In the less condensed metaphases, the telomeric signals could be detected at the end of the euchromatic segment of the duplicated short arm.

The healing of chromosome ends, i.e., the addition of telomere sequences to the broken chromosome ends, has been observed in diverse plant species. In wheat, FISH telomeric signals were detected at the broken ends of deleted chromosomes and at the centromeric regions of telocentric chromosomes [52, 53]. The expression of telomerase has been reported for diverse plant tissues, such as the meristematic tissue and suspension cell cultures [54]. In barley, there was a decrease in the number of telomeric sequences in differentiated cells, and the number of telomeric sequences increased in callus cultures [55]. High telomerase activity was observed in calli derived from tobacco plants, while in leaves the activity was very low [56]. In wheat, during the divisions of the gametophyte, dicentric chromosomes undergo BFB cycles. De novo addition of telomere sequences occurs gradually during the early mitotic divisions in the sporophyte [57].

The present study showing the telomere healing of the broken short arm of chromosome 7 gives evidence of telomerase expression in maize callus culture. The addition of telomeric repeats occurred on a euchromatic region, which was certainly non-telomeric.

The meiosis of the regenerated plants heterozygous for the Df-Dp chromosome 7 was normal. The terminal euchromatic segment was clearly observed at pachytene stage on the duplicated short arm. In the diplotene and diakinesis stages, a heteromorphic pair corresponding to chromosome 7 was observed, as expected for heterozygotes bearing a duplication [9].

2.3 Chromosome 7 and 9 abnormalities in long-term subcultures

C-banded metaphases of subcultures prepared after 18 months of the initiation of the 3–57 callus culture were analyzed during a cultivation period from the 18-month-old original culture to 42-month-old cell lines. The subcultures were designated as cell lines 1-MS2, 2-MS-2, 1-MS1, 2-MS1, 1 N6, and 2 N6. Feulgen-stained anaphases were also observed.

The investigation of mitotic instability by the analysis of Feulgen-stained anaphases showed abnormalities similar to those previously described [8] and shown in **Figure 3**: (i) bridges resulting from delayed chromatids held together at knob sites (**Figure 3A**), (ii) broken bridges (**Figure 3B**), (iii) typical bridges (**Figure 3C, D**), and (iv) fragments (not shown) [9]. The analysis of the frequency of these abnormalities showed a tendency of decreasing frequency with time in culture. Three samples of each cell line were harvested in different periods of cultivation, except 1-MS1 from which seven samples were analyzed. The frequency of anaphase abnormalities observed varied from 4 to 10% in the first sample and from 0.67 to 5.33% in the last sample. This tendency of decreasing frequency was a consequence of the healing of the broken chromosomes, therefore, avoiding an accumulation of BFB cycles [9], as discussed below. Interestingly, the total frequency of abnormalities varied from 0.67 to 10%, and this result was quite similar to the ones observed in a previous study of 5-month-old cultures derived from related inbred lines [38].

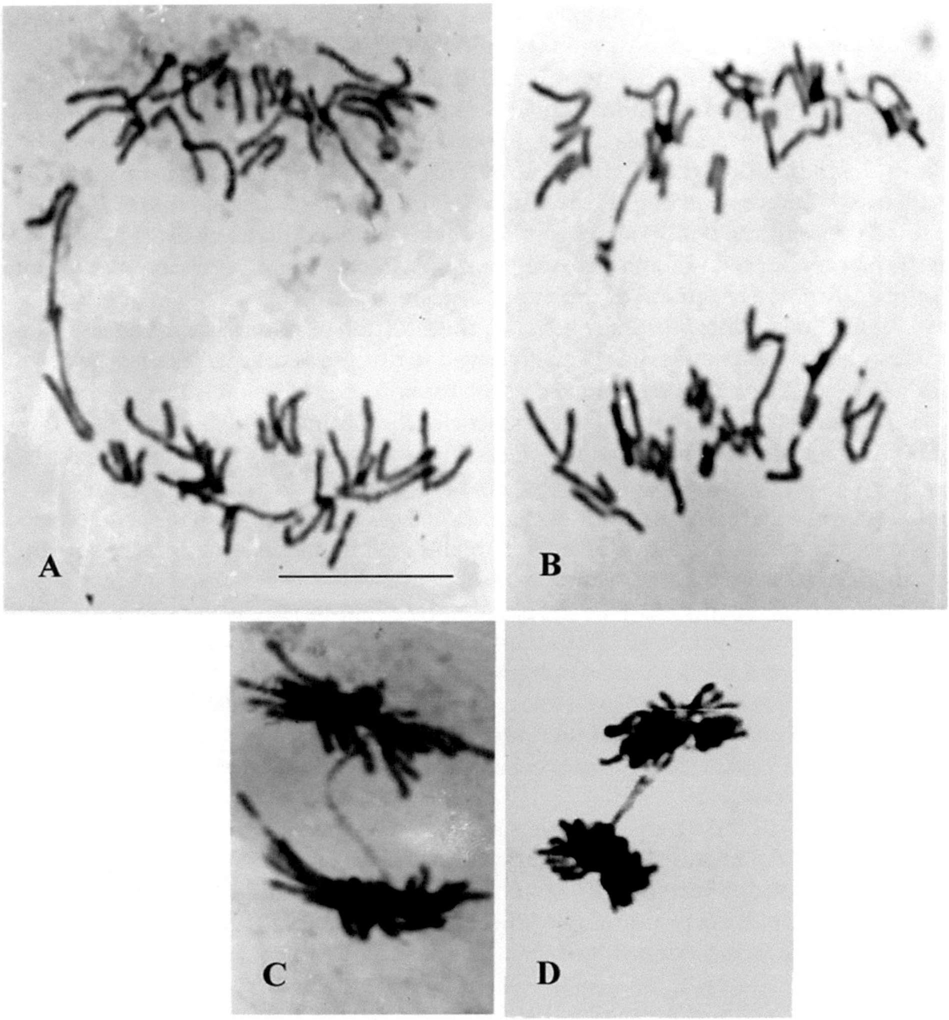

Figure 3.
Feulgen-stained anaphase cells of the cell lines derived from the culture 3–57, with a laggard chromosome showing delayed separating chromatids (A), broken bridge (after the primary event) (B), typical bridge (C), and double bridge (D). Scale bar = 10 μm [9].

The analysis of the cell line pedigree showing the types of chromosomes 7 and 9 observed in C-banded metaphases in different subcultures of the six cell lines is displayed in **Figure 4** [9, 25]. A karyotype diversity among cell lines was detected in this analysis, but homogeneity within some of them was observed in samples harvested at different age transfers. Then, new abnormal chromosomes were stable in different subcultures. Gross aberrations were not observed in chromosomes 6 and 8 that possess knobs smaller than those found in chromosomes 7 and 9.

Different types of abnormal chromosomes 7 and 9 were observed in the cell lines. In the original 18-month-old callus culture 3–57, two types of chromosome 7 were detected. One of the chromosomes possessed two knobs on the short arm (K7S) corresponding to the Df-Dp chromosome 7 described above, and the other type possessed K7S on an interstitial position of a duplicated short arm (**Figure 4**). This chromosome would have originated from a mechanism similar to that shown in

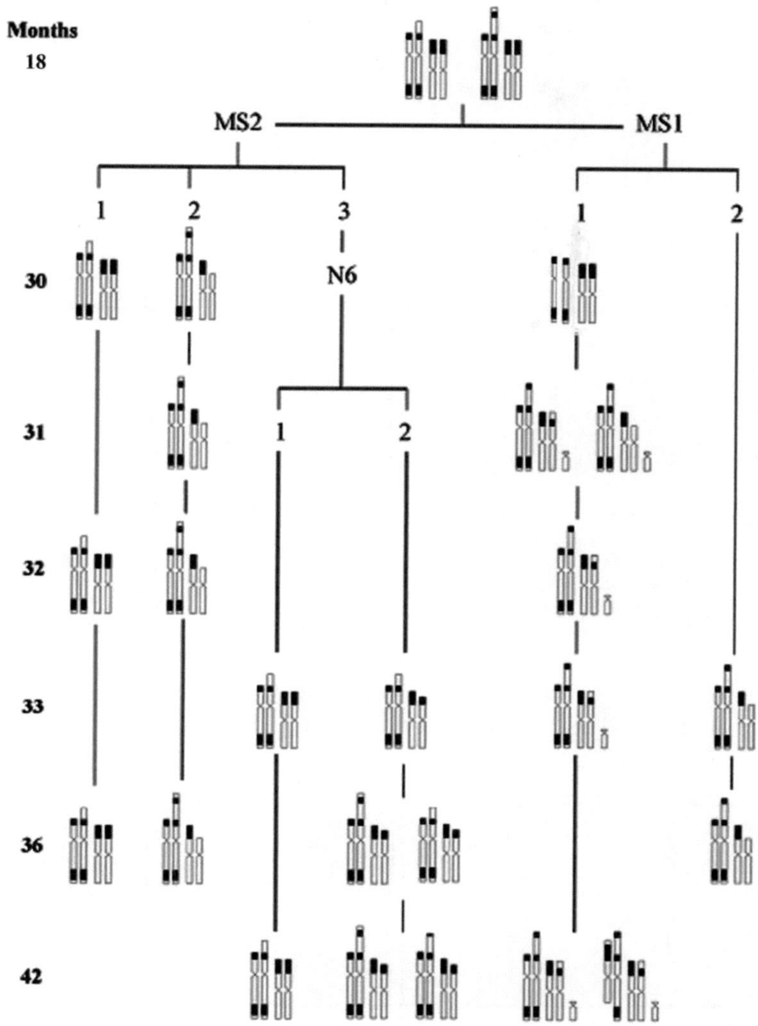

Figure 4.
Cell line pedigree showing the types of chromosomes 7 and 9 observed in C-banded metaphases in different subcultures of the six cell lines derived from culture 3–57 [9, 25].

Figure 1 [9, 25]. The following types of chromosome 7 were distinguished in the cell lines (**Figure 5A**): 7A, normal type, with a terminal K7S and a subterminal K7L; 7B, with a duplicated short arm and a subterminal K7S; 7C, with two knobs on the short arm and a terminal euchromatic segment (similar to **Figure 2B**); 7D, similar to 7C, but without the terminal euchromatic segment; 7E, similar to 7D, with a smaller deficient and terminal K7S; 7F, with a larger short arm, a very large interstitial K7S and without the K7L on the long arm. The 7A, 7B, and 7C types were found in the original 18-month-old culture (**Figure 4**). **Figure 5B**, **C** illustrates the 7D and 7B types, respectively, and the 7E type can be seen in **Figure 5D**. **Figure 5E** illustrates the 7C chromosome. The 7F type can be seen in the pedigree of the 1-MS1 cell line (42-month-old culture, **Figure 6**) [9].

Different types of altered chromosome 9 were also observed in the samples of cell lines (**Figure 5A**) [9]: the normal type corresponds to 9A; a smaller terminal K9S corresponds to 9B; a smaller subterminal K9S corresponds to 9C; 9D is a chromosome without the knob; and 9E is a minichromosome derived from chromosome 9.

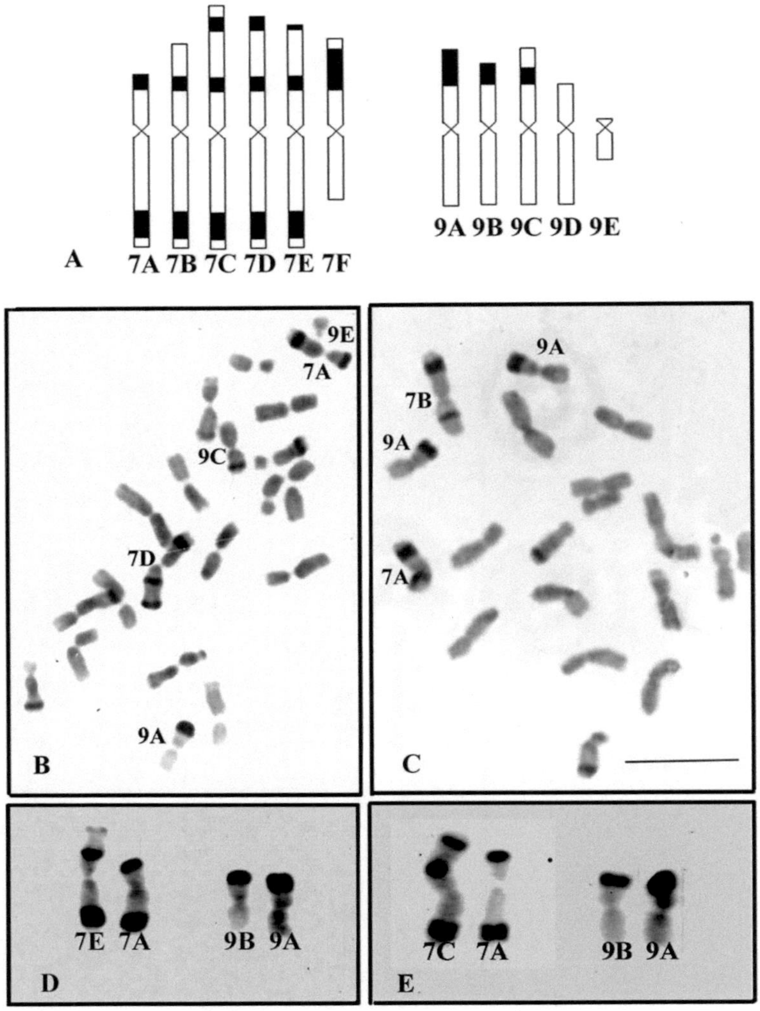

Figure 5.
Types of chromosomes 7 and 9 observed in C-banded metaphase of the cell lines from culture 3–57 (A); metaphase cells of the 1-MS1 cell line (B) and 1MS2 (C); chromosomes 7 and 9 of the N6 cell line(D, E). Scale bar = 10 µm [9, 25].

The 9A, 9C, and 9E types can be seen in **Figure 5B**, and the 9B type is shown in **Figure 5D, E. Figure 6** shows the 9D type, which appears in the 31-month-old subculture of the 1-MS1 cell line. This figure illustrates the different types of chromosomes 7 and 9 detected in 1-MS1 cell line [9, 25].

Therefore, the analysis of metaphases of the cell lines showed new abnormalities in chromosomes 7 and 9. The occurrence of delayed chromatid separation and bridges in anaphases provided evidence of BFB cycle events, and healing of the broken chromosomes could be inferred by the stability of the same abnormal chromosome in different subcultures of the same cell line [9, 25].

In most cell lines, the original abnormal chromosomes 7 (7B and 9C types) were maintained. The 7E type (with a smaller distal K7S) was found in the 42-month-old subculture of the 2-N6 cell line (see **Figure 4**) [9, 25]. The 7D type (chromosome 7 without the terminal euchromatic segment) was observed in the 1-MS1 and 2-MS1. These data suggest that cells bearing the original Df-Dp chromosome 7 (7B or 7C types) were highly adapted in culture and that the new types (7D and 7E) found in

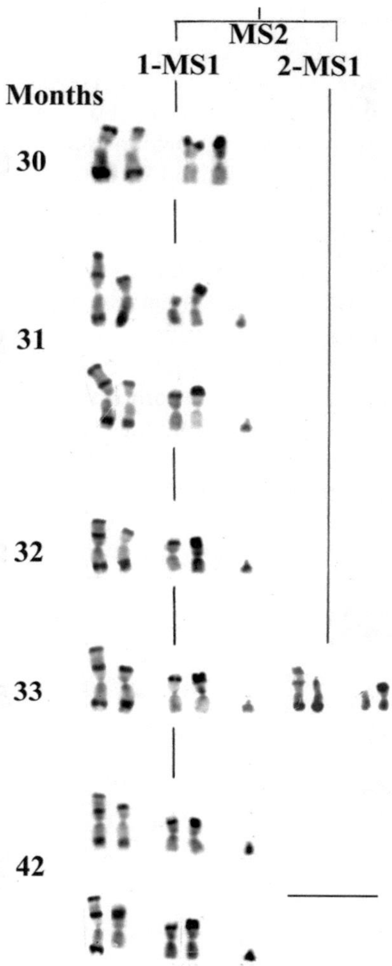

Figure 6.
Types of chromosomes 7 and 9 observed in C-banded metaphases of the 1-MS1 and 2-MS1 cell lines. Scale bar = 10 μm [9].

some subcultures were derived from the original altered chromosome 7 (7C type) through new events of delayed chromatid separation at the knob region and breakage. The 7F type would be a new alteration of the normal chromosome and was detected in the 42-month-old subculture of the 1-MS1 cell line (**Figures 4, 6**) [9, 25]. Its origin would be through a delay in sister chromatids on K7S at anaphase, and an amplified subterminal knob would appear if the duplicate knob did not separate and a breakage occurred at an adjacent euchromatic region. A delayed separation of chromatids on K7L at anaphase, followed by breakage, would explain the absence of this knob in the 7F type.

Chromosome 9 suffered alterations in most cell lines, except for the 1-MS2 and 1-N6 cell lines. The 9D type (K9S deleted) was detected in the 2-MS2 and 2-MS1 cell lines, and the 9B type (partial deletion of the knob) was observed in the 2-N6 cell line (see **Figure 4** [9, 25]). A total or partial deletion of K9S would have occurred after a delay of separation of the chromatids on this knob region and breakage totally or partially eliminating the knob or a segment of it. Interestingly, in the cell line 1-MS1, two types of chromosome 9 appeared, the 9C displaying a subterminal smaller K9S (9C type) and a chromosome without the knob (9D type).

In addition, a minichromosome (9E type) appeared in the subcultures possessing one of these abnormal types. These abnormalities could have resulted from the mechanism suggested in **Figure** 7 [9, 25]. The primary event would be a delay in the separation of chromatids at K9S region followed by breakage originating a deficient knob. Then, two types of BFB cycles, the chromosome [58] and the chromatid types, would have originated the 9C, 9D, and 9E chromosome types. The 9C and 9E chromosome types were observed in several subcultures, thus providing evidence of healing of the broken chromosome ends. In the cell lines analyzed, abnormalities were detected only in chromosomes 7 and 9. These alterations were derived from a primary event of chromatid delayed separation at knob sites in anaphases, followed by breakage and BFB cycle. The presence of large knobs in these chromosomes would lead to this kind of primary event. A case of elimination of chromosome segments from knobbed chromosomes was reported by Rhoades and Dempsey [59]. In the presence of B chromosomes, a bridge formation would occur due to delayed replication of the knob at the second microspore division. Chromosomes containing large knobs would be involved more frequently in this kind of event.

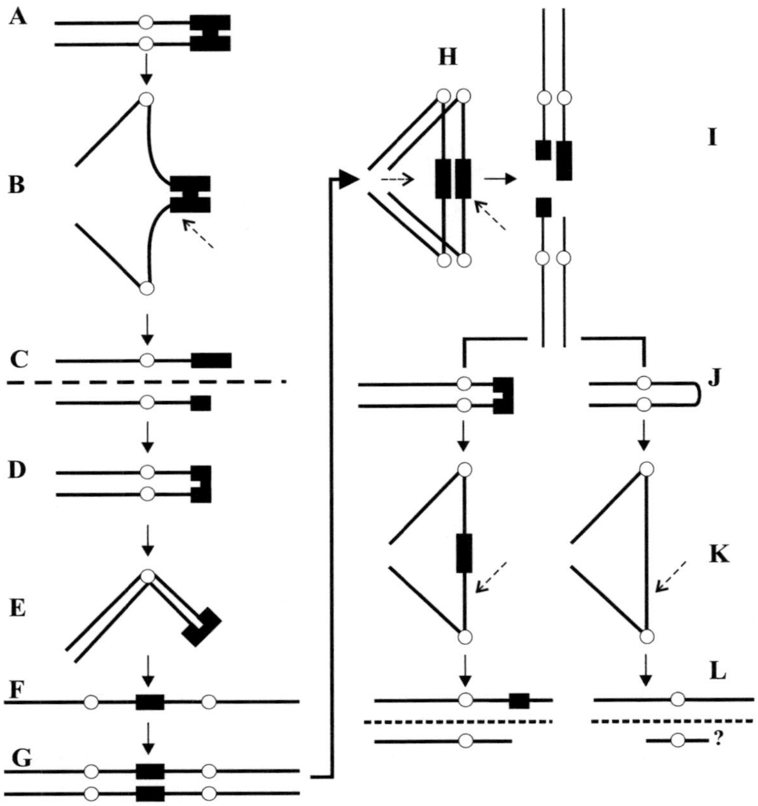

Figure 7.
Mechanism that would originate different types of chromosome 9 in the 1-MS1 cell line: Normal chromosome (A); anaphase with delayed separating chromatids and breakage (B); the resulting chromatids, one normal and the other with a deficient knob (C) fused after replication (D); nondisjunction of sister chromatids (E) resulting in a dicentric chromosome (F, G); double bridge (H) giving rise to a chromatid with a deficiency at K9S and another chromatid without knob (I), which after duplication and fusion (J) suffered breakage in the next anaphases (K); resultant chromosomes: One with a deficient K9S, another without the knob, and a minichromosome originated after deletions whose mechanism is unclear (L). Arrows at anaphases indicate breakpoints [9, 25].

2.4 Heterochromatic knob amplification resulting from unequal crossing over and BFB cycle

The observation of mitotic and meiotic aspects of an amplification of the knob localized on the long arm of chromosome 7 (K7L), in plants regenerated from a long-term callus culture designated 12-F, was carried out aiming to investigate the origin of this amplification. The 12-F original culture was 28 months old when the R1 plants were obtained [10]. The original callus 12-F was heterozygous for the amplified K7L. Therefore, segregation was expected in R_1 progenies derived by selfing R_0 plants. Plants homozygous for the normal and amplified K7L, and plants heterozygous for the amplified K7L, were recovered (**Figure 8**) [10]. The frequency of plants homozygous for the amplification was lower than expected according to Mendelian segregation, while the frequency of plants homozygous for the normal K7L was higher than expected. The frequency of heterozygotes was according to the expected value.

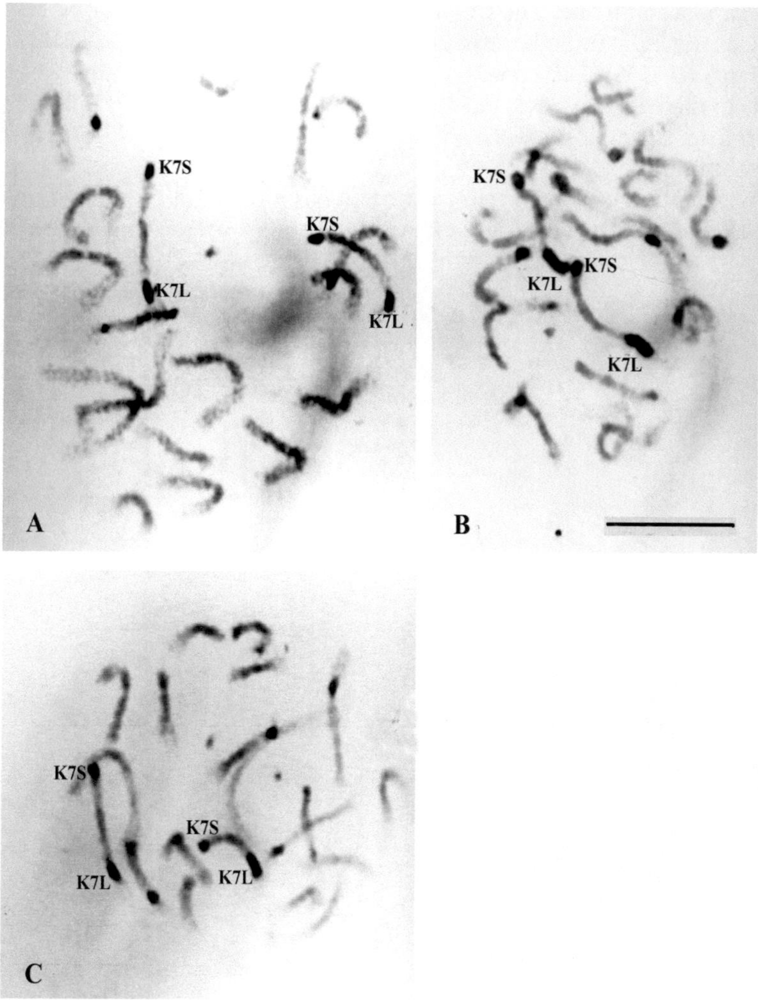

Figure 8.
Somatic chromosomes of regenerated plants (R_1) derived from the 12-F culture: C-banded prometaphase of the homozygote for normal chromosome 7 (A); homozygote for the amplified K7L (B); heterozygote for the amplified K7L (C). Scale bar = 10 μm [10].

Some plants whose karyotype was investigated were selected for meiotic analysis. The homologous chromosomes were completely synapsed on knobs and terminal euchromatic segment on the long arm at pachytene in plants homologous for normal and amplified K7L (**Figure 9A, B**) [10]. In plants heterozygous for the amplification, the knobs and the terminal euchromatic segments were completely synapsed in some cells (**Figure 9C**) [10], but synapsis failure was also detected in these regions (**Figure 9D**) [10]. In chromosomes bearing the K7L amplification and in normal chromosomes, the size of the distal euchromatic segment was similar, but the size of the amplified knob was significantly larger than the normal knob. In a possible case of delay of chromatid separation at this knob site followed by breakage and a BFB cycle, the distal euchromatic segment would be lost as discussed below [10].

Other abnormalities such as translocations, inversions, duplications, and deletions were not found in the chromosomes of these plants derived from a long-term callus culture [10].

The analysis of microsporocytes at the diakinesis stage showed the presence of two types of univalents: one larger with two C-bands, thus corresponding to chromosome 7, and a small one. The frequency of univalents was low for both types. The frequency of the large univalents in heterozygous plants was higher (2.88%) than control plants (0.55%). Differences were not observed in the frequency of small univalents in the heterozygotes (1.14%) in comparison with control plants (1.92%) [10]. Therefore, the meiosis was normal in most microsporocytes, and R2 progenies were also obtained.

The investigation of short-term cultures derived from inbred lines and hybrids related to the inbred line donor of culture 12-F showed interesting alterations on the

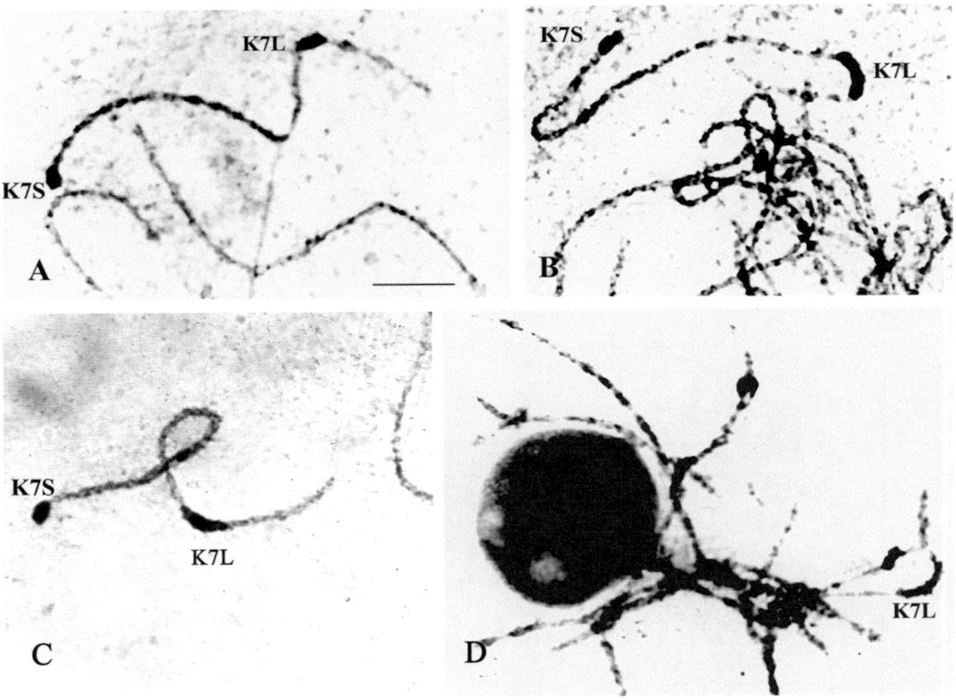

Figure 9.
Carmine-stained meiotic chromosomes of R_1 plants derived from the 12-F culture. Pachytene of a homozygote for the normal K7L (A); homozygote for the amplified K7L (B); heterozygote for the amplified K7L, showing completely synapsed chromosomes (C); pairing failure in the knob region of the heterozygote. Scale bar = 10 μm [10].

long arm of chromosome 7 bearing K7L. The cytogenetic analysis of these cultures detected abnormalities in chromosomes 7 and 9 and other chromosomes with and without knobs. Here we focus only on alterations in the long arm of chromosome 7 to infer the origin of these abnormalities, aiming to understand the origin of the K7L amplification observed in plants derived from culture 12-F. A total of 5223 cells of the callus cultures from 6 genotypes were examined. In three cells from different cultures, chromosome 7 bearing with asymmetric C-bands (corresponding to K7L) was observed: one band was amplified, and the other was reduced in sister chromatids (**Figure 10A, B**). These band alterations would have appeared due to the occurrence of unequal sister chromatid recombination [10].

Unequal crossing over in regions containing duplicate genes or repetitive DNA has been demonstrated in several organisms, such as yeast [60], apes [61], and humans [62]. Two reciprocal products, a directly amplified tandem duplication and a deletion, can result from unequal crossing over between homologous chromosomes. In patients with chromosome duplications involving some types of Charcot–Marie–Tooth disease, the occurrence of unequal recombination between homologous segments (interchromosomal) and sister chromatids (intrachromosomal) has been shown [62]. Thus, the generation of deletions and duplications by unequal recombination can affect the copy number of repeated genes and noncoding repeated DNA sequences.

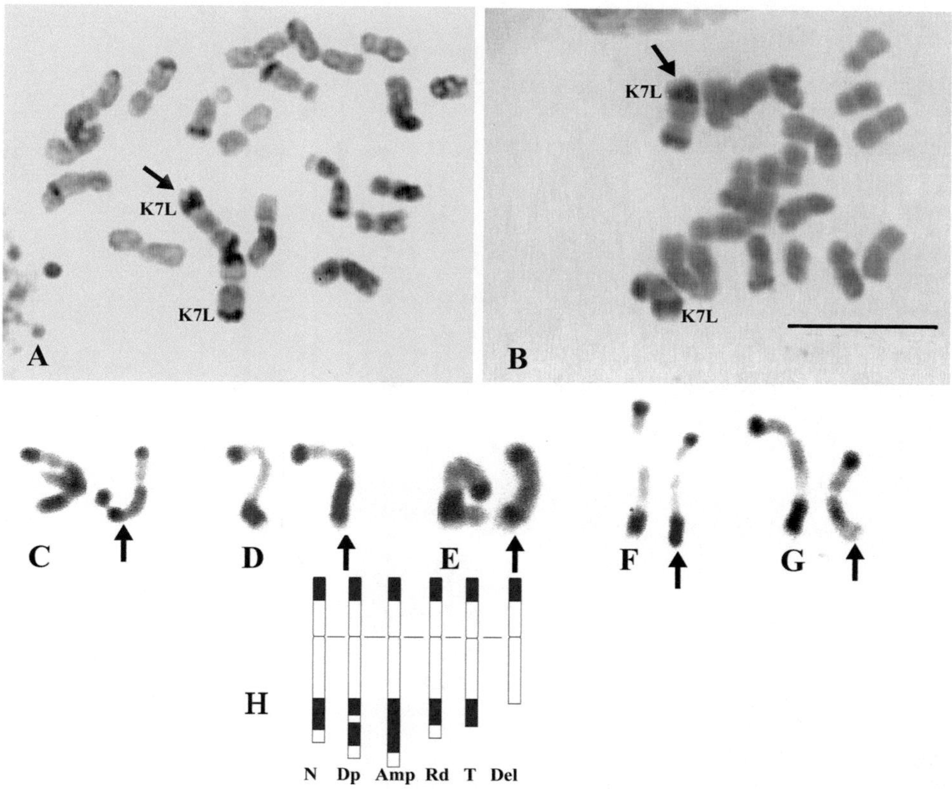

Figure 10.
Types of alterations in the long arm of chromosome 7 observed in C-banded metaphases of the short-term callus cultures: K7L with different sizes in the sister chromatids (A, B); K7L duplication (C); K7L amplification (D); K7L reduction (E); K7L in the telomeric position (F); absence of K7L (G); diagrammatic representation of the abnormal chromosomes (H). Arrows point to the altered chromosomes. N, normal; Dp, duplication; amp, amplification; Rd., reduction; T, terminal; Del, deletion. Scale bar = 10 μm [10].

From this scenario, we can assume that the asymmetric chromosome 7 observed in callus cultures resulted from unequal chromatid recombination at the K7L site. Therefore, the amplification of K7L detected in R1 plants derived from the 12F culture would have originated from an unequal recombination at K7L. This event would not alter the size of the distal euchromatic segment, as observed here [10].

Other alterations were observed on the long arm of chromosome 7 in the callus cultures analyzed: duplication of K7L (**Figure 10C**), amplification of K7L (**Figure 10D**), reduction of K7L (**Figure 10E**), K7L localized on telomeric position (**Figure 10F**), and the absence of K7L (**Figure 10G**). **Figure 10H** shows a diagrammatic representation of these abnormalities. The frequency of these aberrations varied from 0.98 to 4.82% in the six genotypes evaluated [10].

These abnormalities could have originated from a delay of sister chromatid separation at the K7L region, followed by breakage and BFB cycles as suggested in **Figure 11** [10]. After the primary event of delayed chromatid separation, breakage could occur in three different positions at the knob region, terminal (1), proximal (2), and middle (3), giving rise to the different types of abnormalities shown in **Figure 10C–G**. Note that in all possible events, the terminal euchromatic "b" segment would be lost. Regenerated plants homozygous for these aberrations probably would not survive with the deletion of the terminal segment. The recovery of regenerated plants homozygous for the K7L amplification gives support to

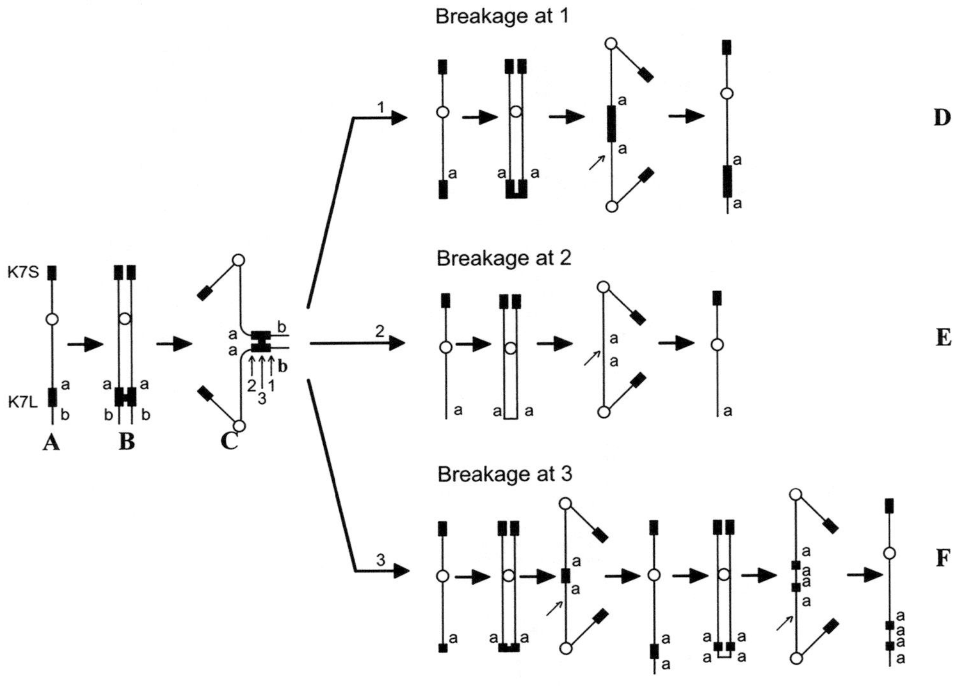

Figure 11.
Diagrammatic representation of the BFB cycles that would result in abnormalities in the long arm of chromosome 7 observed in the short-term callus cultures. The normal chromosome (A) duplicates after DNA replication (B) and delayed separation of the chromatids is observed (C). Breakage occurs at three possible positions: Terminal (1), proximal (2), and middle (3). The resulting chromatids are the following: Breakage at position 1 originates a chromatid with a terminal knob or an amplified knob after a new mitotic cycle (D); breakage at position 2 results in chromatids with the absence of the knob (E); breakage at position 3 results in a reduced terminal knob after the primary event, in a reduced knob and a terminal euchromatic segment after a new mitotic cycle or a duplicated knob after a third mitotic cycle (F). "A" and "b" represent segments near the knobs at a proximal and at a distal position, respectively. Note that in all events, the "b" segment is lost [10].

the hypothesis that this amplification was originated from an unequal chromatid amplification.

Therefore, the results show that knob amplification or reduction can appear as a result of BFB cycles or unequal crossing over, but if they are originated from BFB cycles, they would not survive in homozygous regenerated plants.

3. Conclusions

The presence of some chromosome abnormalities in maize callus cultures can be explained by the occurrence of delay of chromatid separation in mitotic anaphases. This primary event gives origin to a bridge followed by a breakage-fusion-bridge cycle and chromosome healing. FISH using telomere sequences as probes gave evidence of de novo telomere formation at broken chromosome ends. Amplifications and deficiencies in the knobs may also occur via unequal chromosome crossing over evidenced in culture by the presence of chromosome 7 showing differences in the size of K7L (C-band) in sister chromatids.

The data suggest interesting questions for further investigations such as the mechanism underlying the delay in chromatid separation at knob sites and that of de novo telomere formation at the broken chromosome ends in callus culture. Changes in DNA methylation could be the cause of unusual later replication of knobs (see [40]).

The observations on the chromosome healing of chromosomes 7 and 9 showed that this event occurred in euchromatic and heterochromatic regions, certainly non-telomeric sites. Mechanistic information on telomere formation is available through studies on *Saccharomyces cerevisiae*. In this species, telomere sequences were added to non-telomeric broken chromosome ends, but a strong preference for telomerase action was observed at GT, TG, or GG nucleotides [63]. In wheat, de novo telomere formation was initiated by 2-to-4 nucleotide target motifs in an rDNA sequence localized in terminal position [53]. Homologous recombination, nonhomologous end joining, and de novo telomere formation are different mechanisms that repair DNA double strand. De novo telomere formation would be a rare event [64]. In the present report, the healing of chromosomes 7 and 9 possibly occurred in the presence of internal sequences to which telomerase was recruited.

In conclusion, mechanisms of chromosomal evolution like the related here might occur in plants. It has been suggested that structural chromosomal rearrangements frequently appear in euchromatin-heterochromatin borders [65].

Acknowledgements

The authors acknowledge: Canadian Science Publishing for the permission to use figures and data of the article [9]. S. Karger AG for the permission to use figures and data of the article [10]. Nova Science Publishers Inc. for the permission to use figures and data of the review [25]. Fundação de Amparo à Pesquisa do Estado de São Paulo (FAPESP) for research support.

Conflict of interest

The authors declare no conflict of interest.

Author details

Margarida L.R. Aguiar-Perecin[1*], Janay A. Santos-Serejo[2], José R. Gardingo[3] and Mateus Mondin[1]

1 Department of Genetics, Luiz de Queiroz Agriculture College, University of São Paulo, Piracicaba, SP, Brazil

2 Embrapa Cassava and Fruits, Brazilian Agricultural Research Corporation, Cruz das Almas, BA, Brazil

3 University of Ponta Grossa, Ponta Grossa, PR, Brazil

*Address all correspondence to: mlrapere@usp.br

References

[1] McClintock B. Chromosome morphology in Zea mays. Science. 1929;**69**:629-630

[2] Longley AE. Knob position on corn chromosomes. Journal of Agricultural Research. 1939;**59**:475-490

[3] Rhoades MM. Meiosis in maize. Journal of Heredity. 1950;**41**:58-67

[4] Dempsey E. Traditional analysis of maize pachytene chromosomes. In: Freeling M, Walbot V, editors. The Maize Handbook. New York: Spring Verlag; 1994. pp. 432-441

[5] Neuffer MG, Coe EH, Wessler SR. Mutants of Maize. New York: Cold Spring Harbor Laboratory Press; 1997. p. 468

[6] Rhoades MM. Genetic effects of heterochromatin in maize. In: Walden DB, editor. Maize Breeding and Genetics. New York: John Wiley & Sons; 1978. pp. 641-671

[7] Maize Genetics Cooperation Stock Center. Available from: www.maizegdb.org

[8] Fluminhan A, Aguiar-Perecin MLR, Santos JA. Evidence for heterochromatin involvement in chromosome breakage in maize callus culture. Annals of Botany. 1996;**78**:73-81. DOI: 10.1006/anbo.1996.0098

[9] Santos-Serejo JA, Aguiar-Perecin MLR. Breakage-fusion-bridge cycles and de novo telomere formation on broken chromosomes in maize callus cultures. Genome. 2016;**59**:367-378. DOI: 10.1139/gen-2015-0211

[10] Santos-Serejo JA, Gardingo JR, Mondin M, Aguiar-Perecin MLRA. Alterations in heterochromatic knobs in maize callus culture by breakage-fusion-bridge cycle and unequal crossing over. Cytogenetic and Genome Research. 2018;**154**:107-118. DOI: 10.1159/000488067

[11] Aguiar-Perecin MLR, Vosa CG. C-banding in maize II. Identification of somatic chromosomes. Heredity. 1985;**54**:37-42. DOI: 10.1038/hyd.1985.6

[12] Ananiev EV, Phillips RL, Rines HW. A knob-associated tandem repeat in maize capable of forming fold-back DNA segments: Are chromosome knobs megatransposons? Proceedings of the National Academy of Sciences of the United States of America. 1998;**95**:10785-10790. DOI: 10.1073/pnas.95.18.10785

[13] Chen CC, Chen CM, Hsu FC, Wang CJ, Yang JT, Kao YY. The pachytene chromosomes of maize as revealed by fluorescence *in situ* hybridization with repetitive DNA sequences. Theoretical and Applied Genetics. 2000;**101**:30-36. DOI: 10.1007/s001220051445

[14] Page BT, Wanous MK, Birchler JA. Characterization of maize chromosome 4 centromeric sequence: Evidence for an evolutionary relationship with B chromosome centromere. Genetics. 2001;**159**:291-302

[15] Zhong CX, Marshall JB, Topp C, Mroczek R, Nagaki K, et al. Centromeric retroelements and satellites interact with maize kinetochore protein $CENH_3$. Plant Cell. 2002;**14**:2825-2836. DOI: 10.1105/tpc.006106

[16] Nagaki K, Song J, Stupar SM, Parokonny AS, Yuan Q, Ouyang S, et al. Molecular and cytological analyses of large tracks of centromeric DNA reveal the structure and evolutionary dynamics of maize centromeres. Genetics. 2003;**163**:759-770

[17] Kato A, Lamb JC, Birchler JA. Chromosome painting using repetitive

DNA sequences as probes for somatic chromosome identification in maize. Proceedings of the National Academy of Sciences of the United States of America. 2004;**101**:13554-13559. DOI: 10.1073/pnas.0403659101

[18] Albert PS, Gao Z, Danilova TV, Birchler JA. Diversity of chromosomal karyotypes in maize and its relatives. Cytogenetic and Genome Research. 2010;**129**:6-16. DOI: 10.1159/000314342

[19] Ghaffari R, Cannon EKS, Kanizay LB, Lawrence CJ, Dawe RK. Maize chromosomal knobs are located in gene dense areas and suppress local recombination. Chromosoma. 2013;**122**:67-75. DOI: 10.1007/s00412-012-0391-8

[20] Mondin M, Santos-Serejo JA, Bertão MR, Laborda P, Pizzaia D, Aguiar-Perecin MLR. Karyotype variability in tropical maize sister lines and hybrids compared with KYS standard line. Frontiers in Plant Science. 2014;**5**:544. DOI: 10.3389/fpls.2014.00544

[21] Carlson WR. The cytogenetics of corn. In: Sprague GF, Dudley JW, editors. Corn and Corn Improvement. Madison: American Society of Agronomy; 1988. pp. 259-343

[22] Birchler JA, Auger DL, Kato A. Cytogenetics of corn. In: Smith CW, editor. Corn: Origin, History, Technology and Production. New York: John Wiley & Sons; 2004. pp. 427-459

[23] Birchler JA, Bass HW. Cytogenetics and chromosomal structural diversity. In: Bennetzen JL, Hake S, editors. Maize Handbook-Vol II: Genetics and Genomics. New York: Springer; 2009. pp. 163-177. DOI: 10.1007/978-0-387-77863-1_8

[24] Dawe RK. Maize centromeres and knobs (neocentromeres). In: Bennetzen JL, Hake S, editors. Maize Handbook-Vol I: Genetics and Genomics. New York: Springer; 2009. pp. 239-250. DOI: 10.1007/978-0-387-77863-1_8

[25] Aguiar-Perecin MLR, Santos-Serejo JA, Mondin M. Karyotype variability in maize. In: Gorawala P, Mandhatri S, editors. Agricultural Research Updates. Vol. 24. New York: Nova Science Publishers, Inc; 2018. pp. 1-44

[26] McClintock B. Significance of chromosome constitution in tracing the origin and migration of maize in the Americas. In: Walden DB, editor. Maize Breeding and Genetics. New York: John Wiley & Sons; 1978. pp. 159-184

[27] McClintock B, Kato TA, Blumenschein A. Chromosome Constitution of Races of Maize. Colegio de Postgraduados: Chapingo; 1981. p. 517

[28] Ananiev EV, Phillips RL, Rines HW. Complex structure of knob DNA on maize chromosome 9: Retrotransposon invasion into heterochromatin. Genetics. 1998;**149**:2025-2037

[29] Mroczek RJ, Dawe RK. Distribution of retroelements in centromere and neocentromere of maize. Genetics. 2003;**165**:809-819

[30] Kikudome GY. Studies on the phenomenon of preferential segregation in maize. Genetics. 1959;**44**:815-831

[31] Dawe RK, Hiatt EN. Plant neocentromeres: Fast, focused and driven. Chromosome Research. 2004;**12**:55-669. DOI: 10.1023/B:CHRO.0000036607.74671.db

[32] Buckler ES, Phelps-Durr TL, Buckler CSK, Dawe RK, Doebley JF, Holtsford TP. Meiotic drive of chromosomal knobs reshaped the maize genome. Genetics. 1999;**153**:415-426

[33] Dawe RK, Lowry EG, Gent JI, Stitzer MC, Swentowsky KW, et al. A kinesin-14 motor activates neocentromeres to promote meiotic drive in maize. Cell. 2018;**173**:839-850. DOI: 10.1016/j.cell.2018.03.009

[34] Green CE, Phillips RL. Plant regeneration from tissue cultures of maize. Crop Science. 1975;**15**:417-421

[35] Phillips RL, Sommers DA, Hibberd KA. Cell/tissue culture and *in vitro* manipulation. In: Sprague GF, Dudley JW, editors. Corn and Corn Improvement. 3rd ed. Madison: ASA/CSSA/SSSA; 1988. pp. 345-387

[36] Prioli LM, Silva WJ. Somatic embryogenesis and plant regeneration capacity in tropical maize inbreds. Brazilian Journal of Genetics. 1989;**12**:533-566

[37] Furini A, Jewell DC. Somatic embryogenesis and plant regeneration from immature embryos of tropical and subtropical Zea mays L. genotypes. Maydica. 1994;**39**:155-164

[38] Fluminhan A, Aguiar-Perecin MLR. Embryogenic response and mitotic instability in callus cultures derived from maize inbred lines differing in heterochromatic content of chromosomes. Annals of Botany. 1998;**82**:569-576. DOI: 10.1006/anbo.1998.0710

[39] Lee M, Phillips RL. The chromosomal basis of somaclonal variation. Annual Review of Plant Physiology and Plant Molecular Biology. 1988;**39**:413-437. DOI: 10.1146/annurev.pp.39.060188.002213

[40] Peschke VM, Phillips RL. Genetic implications of somaclonal variation in plants. Advances in Genetics. 1992;**30**:41-75. DOI: 10.1016/S0065-2660(08)60318-1

[41] Larkin PJ, Scowcroft WR. Somaclonal variation-a novel source of variability from cell cultures for plant improvement. Theoretical and Applied Genetics. 1981;**60**:197-214. DOI: 10.1007/BF02342540

[42] Sacristan MD. Karyotypic changes in callus cultures from haploid and diploid plants of *Crepis capillaris* (L.) Wallr. Chromosoma. 1971;**33**:273-283. DOI: 10.1007/BF00284945

[43] Lapitan NLV, Sears RG, Gill BS. Translocations and other karyotypic and other structural changes in wheat x rye hybrids regenerated from tissue culture. Theoretical and Applied Genetics. 1984;**68**:547-554. DOI: 10.1007/BF00285012

[44] Lapitan NLV, Sears RG, Gill BS. Amplification of repeated DNA sequences in wheat x rye hybrids regenerated from tissue culture. Theoretical and Applied Genetics. 1988;**75**:381-388. DOI: 10.1007/BF00276739

[45] Murata M, Orton TJ. Chromosomal structural changes in cultured celery cells. In Vitro Cellular & Developmental Biology: Plant. 1984;**19**:83-89. DOI: 10.1007/BF02621890

[46] Johnson SS, Phillips RL, Rines HW. Possible role of heterochromatin in chromosome breakage induced by tissue culture in oats (*Avena sativa* L.). Genome. 1987;**29**:439-446. DOI: 10.1139/g87-076

[47] Lee M, Phillips RL. Genomic rearrangements in maize induced by tissue culture. Genome. 1987;**29**:122-128. DOI: 10.1139/g87-021

[48] Joachimiack A, Ilnick T, Kowalska A, Przywara L. Chromosome alterations in tissue culture cells of *Allium fistulosum*. Genetica. 1995;**96**:191-198. DOI: 1007/BF01439572

[49] McClintock B. The behavior in successive nuclear divisions of

a chromosome broken at meiosis. Proceedings of the National Academy of Sciences of the United States of America. 1939;**25**:405-416. DOI: 10.1073/pnas.25.8.405

[50] McClintock B. The stability of broken ends of chromosomes in *Zea mays*. Genetics. 1941;**26**:234-282

[51] Lukaszewski AJ. Chromatid and chromosome type breakage-fusion-type cycles in wheat (*Triticum aestivum* L.). Genetics. 1995;**140**:1069-1085

[52] Werner JE, Kota RS, Gill BS, Endo TR. Distribution of telomeric repeats and their role in the healing of broken chromosome ends in wheat. Genome. 1992;**35**:844-848. DOI: 10.1139/g92-128

[53] Tsujimoto H, Usami N, Hasegawa K, Yamada T, Nagaki K, Sasakuma T. De novo synthesis of telomere sequences at the healed breakpoints of wheat deletion chromosomes. Molecular & General Genetics. 1999;**262**:851-856. DOI: 10.1007/soo4380051150

[54] Fitzgerald MS, McKnight TD, Shippen DE. Characterization and developmental patterns of telomerase expression in plants. Proceedings of the National Academy of Sciences of the United States of America. 1996;**93**:14422-14427. DOI: 10.1073/pnas.93.25.14422

[55] Kilian A, Stiff C, Kleinhofs A. Barley telomeres shorten during differentiation but grow in callus culture. Proceedings of the National Academy of Sciences of the United States of America. 1995;**92**:9555-9559. DOI: 10.1073/pnas.92.21.9555

[56] Fajkus J, Fulnecková J, Hulánová M, Berková K, Riha K, Matyásek R. Plant cells express telomerase activity upon transfer to callus culture, without extensively changing telomere lengths. Molecular & General Genetics. 1998;**260**:470-474. DOI: 10.1007/s004380050918

[57] Friebe B, Kynast RG, Zhang P, Qi L, Dhar M, Gill BS. Chromosome healing by addition of telomeric repeats in wheat occurs during the first mitotic divisions of the sporophyte and is a gradual process. Chromosome Research. 2001;**9**:137-146. DOI: 10.1023/A:1009283003903

[58] McClintock B. The fusion of broken ends of chromosomes following nuclear fusion. Proceedings of the National Academy of Sciences of the United States of America. 1942;**28**:458-463. DOI: 10.1073/pnas.28.11.458

[59] Rhoades MM, Dempsey E. Chromatin elimination induced by the B chromosome of maize: I mechanism of loss and the pattern of endosperm variegation. Journal of Heredity. 1973;**64**:12-18

[60] Szostak JW, Wu R. Unequal crossing over in the ribosomal DNA of *Saccharomyces cerevisiae*. Nature. 1980;**284**:426-430

[61] Zimmer EA, Martin SL, Beverley SM, Kan Y, Wilson AC. Rapid duplication and loss of genes coding for α chains of hemoglobin. Proceedings of the National Academy of Sciences of the United States of America. 1980;**77**:2158-2162. DOI: 10.1073/pnas.77.4.2158

[62] Stankiewicz P, Lupski JR. Genome architecture rearrangements and genomic disorders. Trends in Genetics. 2002;**18**:74-82

[63] Ribeyre C, Shore D. Regulation of telomere addition at DNA double –strand breaks. Chromosoma. 2013;**122**:159-173. DOI: 10.1007/s00412-013-0404-2

[64] Lamb JC, Shakirov EV, Shippen DE. Plant telomeres. In: Bass H, Birchler JA, editors. Plant Cytogenetics: Genome Structure and Chromosome Function. New York: Springer; 2012. pp. 143-191

[65] Raskina O, Barber JC, Nevo E, Belyayev A. Repetitive DNA and chromosomalrearrangements:Speciation related events in plant genomes. Cytogenetic and Genome Research. 2008;**120**:351-357. DOI: 10.1159/000121084